Boobin' All Day...
Boobin' All Night

A Gentle Approach To Sleep For Breastfeeding Families

by Meg Nagle

International Board Certified
Lactation Consultant

D0710847

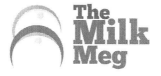
The Milk Meg

www.themilkmeg.com
meg@themilkmeg.com

ISBN: 978-1-511669-41-2

Editor: Erika Hokanson: RefreshMediaResources.com
Cover and comic art: Coral Garvey: coralgarvey.com
Layout and design: Meg Casebolt: caseboltcreative.com

Limit of Liability: My book is not intended to provide medical advice. This publication is for general information only and does not constitute the practice of medicine or replace the advice of your health care provider. What works for one woman might not work for another. Please take what feels right for you and your family and leave the rest behind. Trust your instincts and seek advice from a health care professional as needed.

Praise for Boobin' All Day, Boobin' All Night

Meg tells it like it is – the sweetness and the challenges, without sugar coating. She shares what is normal for the breastfeeding child, why it is important to respond to your child's cues for food and comfort and how you can meet your child's needs and your own, gently and kindly. This is a lovely mix of personal experience, wisdom and the science that validates mothering through breastfeeding – day and night.

-Pinky McKay, IBCLC
author of "Sleeping like a Baby" and "Parenting by Heart"

I love this book! Very personable! It feels like Meg is talking right to me. I wish someone had given this to me for my baby shower. It would have saved me so much wasted time on the internet searching for, 'is it normal that my baby...' when I should have been sleeping! I would have felt so much less alone.

-Devon, breastfeeding mother to Casey

Boobin' All Day, Boobin' All Night is an amazing and informative book. I wish I'd had my hands on this gem when my 16 month old was a newborn. I would not have shed so many tears! Thank you, Meg, for assuring us sleep-deprived, worried mamas that it isn't abnormal for babies & toddlers to wake up for boob at night!

-Nicole, breastfeeding mother to Emily

Meg has put together a remarkable guide to helping raise infants and children in the most natural and healthy way. Her down to earth writing style and content can be understood and applied by any frazzled, sleep deprived parent. I highly recommend this book to all parents. This should be mandatory reading in all parenting classes!

-Aram Kalpakgian, Pediatric Physician's Assistant

While I was pregnant, I read several baby sleep books that put *me* to sleep, because although their advice was well-thought-out, they were really boring to read. Then my son came along and I forgot or ignored most of the advice in those books, because they were way too extreme for how I wanted to take care of my little man.

Meg's book isn't boring, or sterile, or preachy. She's a mother, talking to other mothers, telling them that it's ok to follow their intuition because maternal instinct is a real thing and babies aren't robots who sleep through the night at 8 weeks. This book meets mamas where we are, in the real world.

-Meg, breastfeeding mother to Sam

This book would have saved me a lot of tears and heartache if I had read it 15 years ago with the birth of my first child instead of trying to learn things on my own. Meg combines science with real life experience to give the reader a confidence needed in raising even the most difficult child. I would highly recommend this book to all my friends, and to all parents, doctors, and lactation consultants.

-Michelle, breastfeeding mother to her youngest of five children

Dedication

This book is dedicated to:

My husband who supported me and our little breastfeeders through frequent night-waking to breastfeed, mastitis fire boob, gushing over-supply boobs, breastfeeding a premature baby, co-sleeping, bedsharing, breastfeeding to natural term and complaints of sleep deprivation. You are a gem.

My mother who always spoke about her love of breastfeeding my sister and I, and who twenty years later attempted to relactate for her adopted daughter.

My father who supported my mother while breastfeeding us and for frequently telling me what a great mother I was for breastfeeding my boys.

My most favorite story teller Carla, who spoke frequently of her adventures in parenting, breastfeeding and motherhood.

Deb, my La Leche League leader who taught me so much, helped me become a leader, and continues to support breastfeeding women.

Aram, my first born's Pediatric Physician's Assistant who guided me and supported me through my early years as a new breastfeeding mother. You encouraged me to trust my instincts and your support was just what a new mother needed.

Each and every woman I have ever worked with who taught me more than books or research articles ever could.

My three boys who have taught me how to mother through breastfeeding.

Acknowledgements

A big thank you to Erika, Janine, Carla, Devon, Chris and Erica for your help in the final proofreading/editing stages!

Thank you Meg for all of your help with the design of my book and bringing it all together.

Thank you to Coral for turning my comic ideas into actual drawings (as my own stick figure versions just would not have had the same awesomeness of your drawings) and for the amazing cover art.

Thank you Aishah for all of your help with the publishing side of things! Your insight and knowledge is priceless!

Last but definitely not least, thank you to Diana West, IBCLC for your help with my co-sleeping and bedsharing chapter. I am so happy to be giving mothers the most up-to-date information and resources so they can make informed decisions on how to safely sleep with their breastfed babies.

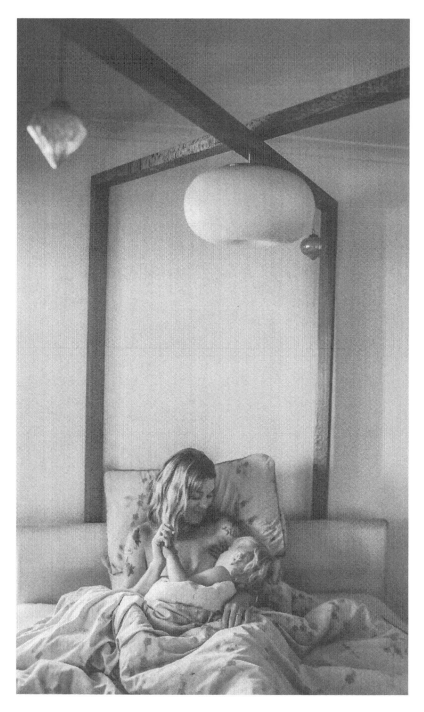

My youngest and I breastfeeding in the most comfortable spot.
Photo Credit: Melissa Jean Photography Australia

Table of Contents

Comics (because all of us sleep deprived mothers need to laugh) and posters (because who doesn't like a poster!?) spread throughout.

Foreword

If you're reading these words, you've been drawn to something intriguing about this book on breastfeeding and sleep. Your instincts were right on target, just as they've likely been throughout your journey of becoming a new parent.

Caring for a baby around the clock can push us to the limit of our skills. It's unrelenting. When a normal job would at least give us time to sleep, baby care continues all night long. As much as we love our babies and want to do the very best we can for them, utter exhaustion can set in quickly if we don't find ways to care for them while we care for ourselves, too.

That's where this wonderful book comes in. Meg has a gentle approach of helping us find ways to honor our baby's important needs as we respect our own basic needs. This book is filled with wonderful ideas and strategies for making both days and nights with your baby more fulfilling and enjoyable. I like that it's realistic, clearly coming from her own lived experience. But it's also grounded in science with the latest understandings of the importance of breastfeeding and infant attachment.

When we're in the darkest hours of the night, whether an actual night or the metaphorical night of new parenthood, this book can be a reassuring and calming voice to help you trust your instincts and listen to your baby. It won't be hard to picture Meg with an arm around your shoulder, quietly reminding you that you're doing a wonderful job. And that you're a member of a wonderful sisterhood of mothers around the world caring for the babies in the small hours of the night, even at this very moment.

Enjoy the delicious words in this beautiful book. May they fill your tired soul with the reassurance, inspiration, and ideas to find the next step on your journey of motherhood.

Diana West, IBCLC
April 15, 2015

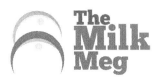

A Boobin' Side Note from Meg...

> *gentle [jen-tl], adjective*
>
> *1. having or showing a mild, kind, or tender temperament or character; "a gentle, sensitive man"*
>
> *synonyms: kind, kindly, tender, benign, humane, lenient, merciful, forgiving, forbearing, sympathetic, considerate, understanding, clement, compassionate, benevolent, kindhearted, tender-hearted, good-natured, sweet-tempered, loving;*
>
> *2. moderate in action, effect, or degree; not strong or violent; "a gentle breeze"*
>
> *synonyms: light, soft, zephyr-like, moderate, pleasant*

This gentle guide to sleep is for breastfeeding mothers out there who are looking for alternatives to cry-it-out or sleep training methods. As a new mother, it did not feel right for me to let my baby cry (even for a short time) but I was also completely exhausted and confused as to what I should do. I know there are millions of you out there who feel the same. Mothering through breastfeeding is something that happens during the day as well as during the night. Babies and toddlers will respond differently to my ideas and suggestions so please try the ones that make sense to you and your family. You may read a section of this book and think I'm right on target and then read the next bit and think I've gone insane! There is no step-by-step guide here because what works for one mother might not work for another, and there are a variety of ways to practice gentle parenting (especially when it comes to sleep).

I've included different possible solutions for sleep challenges that breastfeeding mothers face. Do what works for you and forget about the rest if it doesn't feel right. You are your baby's own baby whisperer and you know your baby best.

A word on "boob"... I love the word "boob" and I get quite tired of the formal, medical terminology ... especially when writing about something we have been doing since the beginning of time, before the medical world even existed. Here in Australia (where I live) many of us say the word "booby" and "boob" frequently! I use the following words interchangeably, just to keep things interesting: breasts, boobs, and boobies. I also use the terms "breastfeeding" and "boobin'" which both simply mean feeding your baby from your breast, or the act of a mother or child breastfeeding. I also use "he" and "she" randomly throughout the book since we have both in the world.

A BABY WAKING
WHEN PUT DOWN
IS NOT A
BABY WITH A
SLEEP PROBLEM.
IT'S A BABY
COMMUNICATING
THAT THEY NEED
SOME CUDDLES.

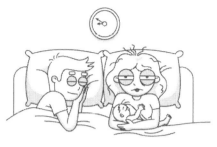

Why Our Breastfed Babies and Toddlers Wake so Frequently

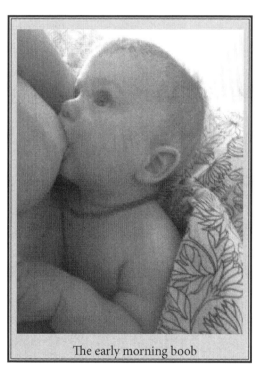
The early morning boob

Regardless of how you feed your baby, there will be moments when you are so sleep deprived you feel as though you are going to go crazy. That feeling that you get being woken up just after you finally got back to sleep, waking every hour on a particularly bad night where your nipple was in your baby's mouth pretty much the entire time... sleep deprivation is the cruelest form of torture!

So as a breastfeeding mother who is the only person available to feed the baby, how can we get some rest and relaxation while continuing to mother our babies at night through breastfeeding? Why are our babies waking so often and without a predictable pattern?

We all question ourselves and whether we are making the right decisions on how we go about feeding our babies at night. We often ask if it's normal that our babies are waking so often and if we will ever get more than one or two hours straight of sleep?! The answer to both questions is YES!

Many of us are told by our family members or friends at our baby's playgroup that our baby should be sleeping through. We hear stories from other mothers about how their little ones have been sleeping through for weeks or months and everyone looks at you with pity in their eyes and surprise that your strange little baby is still waking. We almost feel like alien mothers who have a problem child on our hands. We are told that our babies really need to learn how to sleep on their own and NEED to know how to self-settle and get through the night without relying on us and our boobs.

My philosophy as an International Board Certified Lactation Consultant and mother of three (currently feeding my youngest as I write this sentence) is that it's important to discuss WHY our babies and toddlers wake throughout the night and stress that it's not only the biological norm for this to happen, but it's actually really important for many reasons.

*Let me take a moment to bring up a very important point. Many times I have been asked, "My baby sleeps through the night! Is that OK?" There is nothing wrong with your baby if they sleep for long periods of time! Do a little dance and pat yourself on the back for having a baby who likes to sleep! Some breastfed babies and toddlers sleep for long chunks and there is nothing wrong with that. Go put your feet up and drink a cup of tea! Oh yes, and I kind of hate you right now.

Why most breastfed babies and toddlers wake frequently to breastfeed:

Research shows that frequent night-waking to breastfeed is a protective factor against SIDS. "Many researchers believe that arousal deficiency—the inability of an infant to arouse and breathe following an otherwise normal breathing pause or apnea—may play an important role in the etiology of SIDS.

If this is true, then manipulation of the conditions that facilitate arousability might be protective against SIDS. This might be especially true during quiet sleep (Stages 1–4) given the relatively low rate of spontaneous arousals generally associated with this sleep stage and especially the relatively high arousal threshold required to arouse from deep (Stages 3–4) sleep."[1] So more frequent waking (which is what breastfed babies tend to do) is actually a positive thing! They arouse easily from sleep to breastfeed which in turn helps to decrease the likelihood of SIDS.

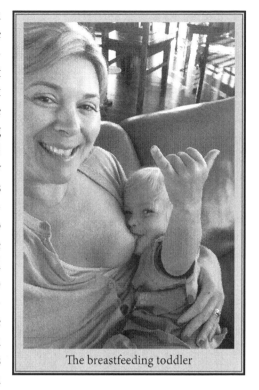

The breastfeeding toddler

Frequent night-waking helps establish and keep up your milk supply. Research shows that babies take up to 20 percent of their milk volume at night.[22] Sleep-training and cry-it-out techniques can decrease your milk supply. Mothers who are told to ignore their babies' cries in some instances will find it more difficult to be responsive to their infants in other instances. This is a case of culture overriding a mother's hardwired response to her baby. Spacing out feedings and/or stopping night feedings at some arbitrary age will have a direct impact on her milk supply, opening the door to milk-supply issues, decreased weight gain,

1. McKenna J, McDade, T. Why babies should never sleep alone: A review of the co-sleeping controversy in relation to SIDS, bedsharing and breastfeeding. *Paediatric respiratory reviews.* 2005; 6, 134-152.

2. Kent JC, et al. Volume and frequency of breastfeedings and fat content of breast milk throughout the day. *Pediatrics.* 2006; 117(3):387-395.

increased supplementation, and possibly failure to thrive.[3] For some women, especially in the early months or years, if they are going to be separated from the baby or toddler during the day, these night-time feedings will be crucial for keeping up breastmilk supply. This helps especially for women who are returning to work and are worried about their supply. Night feeding can take away much of that worry.

Although we all make the same amount of milk within a 24-hour period, we have different storage capacities. This means that for some babies, breastfeeding frequently will be absolutely crucial for getting the milk they need to be nourished and to grow. Some babies can go three or four hours between breastfeeding, others will breastfeed every hour. In a study from Konner 2006, it was found that the traditional feeding pattern of babies from the !Kung tribe of South Africa, was to breastfeed very quickly, but frequently (about 4 times per hour).[4] My own conversations with women the last decade (and my own personal experiences) have shown me that for women who breastfeed following their babies' cues, most often the babies breastfeed quite frequently at times in a bit of a cyclical fashion over the weeks and months. Sometimes they feed a few times per hour, day and night. These cycles can last hours, days, or sometimes months before changing to a different spacing pattern.

Babies will wake more frequently when they are going through a growth spurt and need to increase your supply, are going through a developmental milestone, teething, or are fighting an illness they have been exposed to. Many times women will be holding their eyelids open with toothpicks from the night before, only to discover that later that day their baby is

---

3. Kendall–Tackett, K. Why Cry-It-Out And Sleep Training Techniques Are Bad For Babes. *Clinical Lactation.* http://www.clinicallactation.org/sites/default/files/articlepdf/CL4-2Editorial.pdf Published 2013. Accessed November 2, 2014.

4. Konner M. Hunter-gatherer infancy and childhood: The !Kung and others. In: BS Hewlett and ME Lamb, eds. *Hunter-gatherer childhoods: Evolutionary, developmental and cultural perpectives.* New Brunswick: Transaction Publishers; 2005. http://www.parentingscience.com/infant-feeding-schedule.html#sthash.yMzNDdzR.dpuf

coughing and has a stuffy nose! It's a wonderful feeling knowing that their needs have been met through breastfeeding and that makes the sleep deprivation so worth it.

Research shows that the growth of our babies' brains (DNA synthesis) happens rapidly during the first few years of life, along with nerve growth factors including a hormone that facilitates development. These are both promoted through touch, and when mothers stop touching their infants, DNA synthesis stops and the growth hormone diminishes.[5] When our babies are put down and left by themselves as they cry in distress, they go into survival mode.[6]**Breastmilk has components that help our babies and toddlers fall asleep.**[7]**It's like a natural sleep aid!** This is why it is the biological norm for babies and toddlers to fall asleep while breastfeeding. Your baby does not have a sleep problem because they will not self-settle or fall asleep on their own in a cot. Your milk is literally made to help them fall asleep while breastfeeding. It is how our bodies are designed. So cool! No crying involved, just pop them on! The only way a baby can communicate is through crying. A research article published in 2011[8]showed that although babies stopped crying on about the third night after sleep-training, the level of the stress hormone cortisol was still raised. Even though they had been trained to fall asleep and were quiet and seemingly peaceful, they still had elevated stress hormones within their body. This is a physiological response that was recorded and shows just how distressing it is for a baby, even when they are sleeping after a cry-it-out experience.

---

5. Schanberg S. The genetic basis for touch effects. In Field T, ed. *Touch and Early Experience*, Mahwah, NJ: Erlbaum. 1995.

6. Narvaez, D. How To Grow A Smart Baby. *Psychology Today.* http://www. psychologytoday.com/blog/moral-landscapes/201101/how-grow-smart-baby. Published January 24, 2011. Accessed November 11, 2014.

7. Sánchez C, et al. The possible role of human milk nucleotides as sleep inducers. *Nutritional Neuroscience.* 2009; 12, 2-8.

8. Middlemiss W, Granger D, Goldberg W, Nathans L. Asynchrony of mother–infant hypothalamic–pituitary–adrenal axis activity following extinction of infant crying responses induced during the transition to sleep. *Early Human Development.* 2012; 88, 227-232.

We often forget that babies and toddlers wake for many reasons other than hunger. They will of course wake for hunger or thirst but they will also wake for pain relief, comfort, to get an increase in the immunological components in breastmilk, to help them cope with their developmental milestone and the changes in their brain due to this, or if they are scared, cranky, or bored!

There are many sleep-training articles and websites that state that if your baby or toddler is sleeping through the night they will do better in school, have less chance of being obese, and have an increased ability to learn. These statements are incredibly misleading. There is NO research to support the claim that babies and toddlers who fall asleep at the breast and breastfeed throughout the night are more likely to be overweight, have trouble in school, or have a hard time learning. To create a valid study on this issue, we'd need a longitudinal study that specifically compares those who are exclusively breastfed to sleep and through the night with those who are sleep-trained and night-weaned, leaving out variables that could also affect the results AND have it be peer reviewed. This has not happened yet and therefore any study that is quoted is not valid or relevant to the issue of night waking in babies and toddlers.

So when will my child actually start sleeping through? Doesn't it get harder the older they get? Actually, for many of us we find it gets easier the older they get. Once your child is over the 12-month mark they will understand pretty much everything you are saying. Once they start to communicate more themselves (usually nearing the 18-month mark) it becomes much easier to negotiate night-time weaning with them and becomes less stressful for everyone involved. This is when they are developmentally ready to negotiate and understand what you are saying to them. Before this time, many mums find it incredibly difficult, distressing, and frustrating to try night-weaning. Of course if your baby is younger than this and is responding without crying or distress at falling asleep on her own then great—go with it!

There's no denying that waking overnight to breastfeed and soothe a baby takes a toll on us as mothers. If we can shift our thinking away from the baby and their sleep issues then we can start focusing on ourselves and what we can change. We tend to run around like crazy in our society… take a deep breath and relax.

Mothering through breastfeeding is one of the most natural, biologically normal things you can do for your child and it meets every single one of their night-time needs. Breastfeeding to sleep, breastfeeding to awake, breastfeeding for hunger, comfort, or pain relief… every reason is important and night-time waking to breastfeed is something that millions of us women do around the world every single night. Trust your instincts and follow the lead of your baby. No mother looks back and feels guilty for cuddling or breastfeeding her baby too often. You cannot spoil a baby. You cannot cuddle them too often, breastfeed them too frequently, or love them too much.

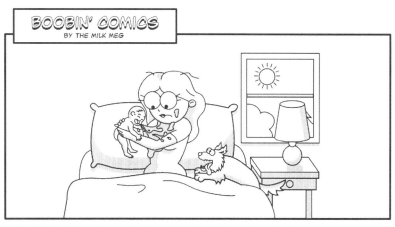

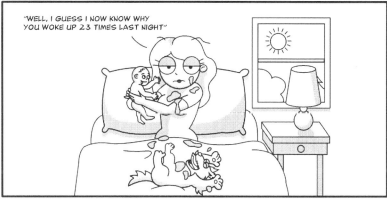

Seven Crucial Steps to Increasing & Maintaining Your Breastmilk Supply

Frequent night-waking helps keep up your supply. Here are some things to focus on if you are worried about your supply.

You cannot overfeed a breastfed baby, BUT in some cases they can be extra sleepy and will need to be woken up.

Hang out with your baby skin-to-skin as often as possible in the early weeks and whenever you feel as though your supply needs a boost.

Breastfeed your baby by following their natural cues... not the clock or the schedule in a book you were given.

Keep On Boobin'

Breastfeed throughout the night to not only help keep your supply up, but also meet your baby's night time needs through breastfeeding.

Sleep near (co-sleeping) or with (bedsharing) your baby following safe guidelines.

Make sure your baby is efficiently sucking and removing your milk.

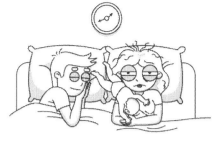

The Milk Meg's Night-Waking Survey

How Many Of Us Have Frequent Night-Wakers?

I am so excited to share the result of my survey. We all want to know if our breastfed child is like everyone else's! So what are women actually experiencing with their breastfed babies when they do not do any sort of sleep-changing or responsive-settling techniques? What about those of us who breastfeed at night as well as during the day? What about toddlers? Isn't it normal for babies but not toddlers?

Now I have to make some things very clear. This was a very simple poll with only three questions. There was only one requirement to take the poll: you had to be breastfeeding, of course! I am not a researcher; I do not do this sort of thing… ever. It's pretty much the first poll I've ever created in my life! I hope this gives some insight into what breastfeeding mothers are experiencing as I received over 8,000 responses total for these three surveys!

The poll was shared on Facebook and I received responses from women around the world. There was no definition of "breastfeeding" so some of these women might be supplementing and might not be breastfeeding on demand. However this makes the results even more awesome because even if this is the case (that some of them are supplementing, bottle feeding here or there, or schedule feeding) the majority of these women have babies and toddlers who are continuing to wake regardless!

Only 8.6% of babies aged 0–12 months and just 6.8% of children aged 13–24 months were sleeping through at the time of taking this poll! That is a very small percentage of women. As expected the percentage of children aged 25+ months who were sleeping through was larger, at about 20%. Yet over 66% were waking 1–3 times and over 12% 4–6 times per night! Many women have breastfeeding toddlers who continue to wake. It's also interesting to note that in both the 0–12 and 13–24 month age groups over 25% of babies and toddlers were waking 4–6 times. That is more than a quarter of them waking to breastfeed quite frequently.

How frequently does your child wake at night?

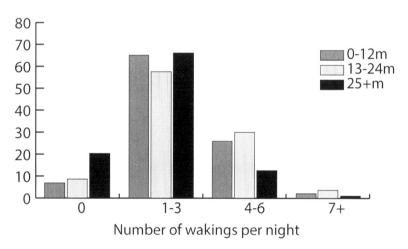

Number of wakings per night

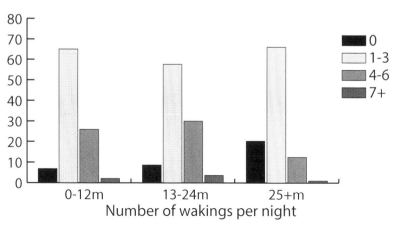

Number of wakings per night

Cluster feeding (feeding on and off very frequently) is something that many baby books mention and is now widely known about, however we often do not realize that cluster feeding might happen at odd times of the day (or night) and will continue beyond babyhood. In my own personal experiences, and the time spent working with other breastfeeding mothers, I have noticed that many of us find our babies and toddlers cluster feeding in the early morning hours leading up to sunrise. I thought this was an important question to ask as I had a feeling that many women would answer "yes" or "sometimes."

Does your baby cluster-feed (breastfeed very frequently) in the early morning hours leading up to sunrise?

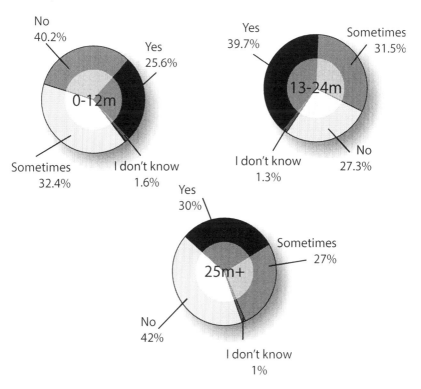

I did a little happy dance when I saw the results because my hypothesis proved to be true in the responses to this question! A larger percentage of babies in the 13–24m and 25+m age groups did early morning cluster feeding than in the 0–12 month age group! Babies do tend to sleep in longer chunks when they are very little, only to start breastfeeding a bit more frequently as they get older. In the 25+ month group, 30% answered "yes" to this question and over 27% answered "sometimes!" So it is not uncommon for toddlers to cluster feed, as well as babies.

This information is so helpful for mothers as their breastfeeding children grow. We often think that as our baby gets older they will cluster feed less and sleep in longer stretches. This is often not the case as our older breastfeeding children continue to cluster feed and it is completely normal… and important!

The final question in my poll was about the pattern of children's night-waking.

How would you describe your child's sleep patterns?

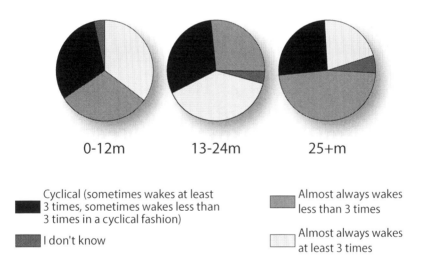

0-12m   13-24m   25+m

Cyclical (sometimes wakes at least 3 times, sometimes wakes less than 3 times in a cyclical fashion)

I don't know

Almost always wakes less than 3 times

Almost always wakes at least 3 times

The cyclical patterns of night-waking are an important aspect of night-time mothering through breastfeeding. Many of us start to see that our babies and toddlers will sleep so well for ages, only to start waking more frequently again for no reason! We try so hard to find a reason, grasping at straws and trying to find answers as to WHY they are waking so frequently after they had such a long stretch of only waking one or two times per night. From working with women for so long and hearing about their experiences with this, I knew that it was something that many of us faced and even more: I knew it was NORMAL!

It's interesting that for this question, the percentages for each answer were very similar between the 0–12m and 13–24m age groups. Even in the 25+m survey, just over 25% of women described their child's night-waking patterns as "cyclical" and 21% selected "Almost always wakes at least three times."

So what does this all mean? Not every breasted baby continues to wake at night beyond babyhood, yet you can see from these results that for many breastfeeding women, babies and toddlers continue to wake throughout the night at least once, tend to cluster feed at least some of the time in the early morning hours, and often have cyclical sleep patterns. Trust your instincts and follow the lead of your child. You are doing a great job! Find mother-to-mother breastfeeding support groups where you can get some words of comfort and understanding from others who mother through breastfeeding at night, just like you.

THERE IS NO NORMAL WHEN IT COMES TO NIGHT WAKING. THE ONLY NORMAL THING ABOUT IT IS THE UNPREDICTABLE NATURE OF THE FREQUENCY AND CAUSE. SLEEPING THROUGH, WAKING ONCE, WAKING TWICE, WAKING SIX TIMES... IT'S ALL NORMAL.

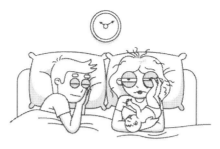

Breastfeeding Your Baby to Sleep... What's the Big Deal?!

I remember a dear friend Erin who had a baby a few months after me. This was way back in time when I was still young and fresh and had only one grey hair instead of ten (OK fine, twenty). This was a few months after my second boy was born. Erin and I hung out quite a bit and realized quickly that we mothered our babies very differently! As I sat there breastfeeding my baby to sleep, Erin would rock and jiggle and burn off the breakfast she just ate, trying to get her baby to sleep. This is because she was trying to keep the strict schedule of feed, play, sleep... or is it sleep, play, feed?! She and many other women out there believed it was not good to let a baby fall asleep at the breast. So as my baby peacefully and happily fell asleep while breastfeeding, her baby was staring

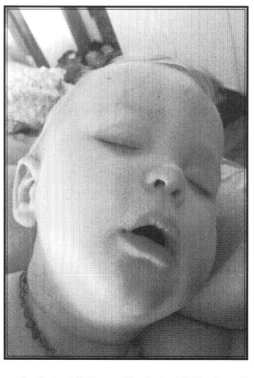

at me with her wide gorgeous eyes as she was being jiggled. Where did this concept come from? Who thought of it in the first place? I'd like to have a word with them.

Believe me, for all of you out there who have trained your baby to fall asleep alone, I understand your frustration. I understand why you went down that road. I understand how difficult the whole sleep issue can be. I just have a different perspective...

First let's look at normal infant behavior...

- Most babies LOVE to be cuddled (doesn't everyone?).
- Most babies LOVE to be comforted when they are upset or tired (doesn't everyone?).
- Most babies would much rather fall asleep with someone next to them instead of by themselves, alone in a big room (wouldn't everyone?).
- Most babies and toddlers would choose to breastfeed to sleep rather than just fall asleep on their own (wouldn't everyone? OK, maybe not past childhood...).

All human babies thrive on touch and our mental and physical wellbeing actually helps build our bond and relationship with our babies. Touching and cuddling happens every time you breastfeed your baby. Touch plays a critical role in parent-child relationships from the start: "It's an essential channel of communication with caregivers for a child," says San Diego State University School of Communication Professor Emeritus Peter Andersen .[1]

Babies are social creatures, just like us! Unless you are a loner who is anti-social and would much rather wander by yourself than go to a party (Dad, I'm talking about you here) then you are a social being. Babies need a lot of social and parental interaction because they are born prematurely compared to other mammals. Instead of asking, "Why should I feed my baby/toddler to sleep?" The question should be, "Why would I do anything BUT

---

1. Chillot R. The power of touch. *Psychology Today.* https://www. psychologytoday.com/articles/201302/the-power-touch Published 11 March, 2013. Accessed 8 December, 2014.

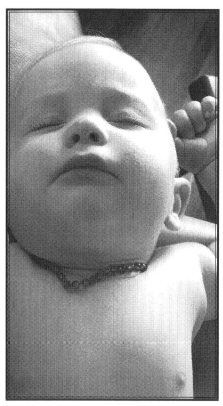

breastfeed my baby/toddler to sleep?" It's the most natural and normal thing in the world! And because babies are social creatures, it would also make sense that when they are active—eating, sleeping, playing, or just plain old hanging out—they want to share those activities with someone! Therefore even the simple practice of falling asleep is actually a social activity. When you think about it, having a baby (yes, even an older baby or toddler) fall aslccp by thcmsclvcs seems quite strange and unnatural.

The composition of breastmilk also has properties that help babies fall asleep. Not only does it nourish and protect our babies, it also helps them to relax. This is not by accident. There are no accidents in nature (well, except my natural progression to dressing like Courtney Love in 8th grade but that's a whole other story which requires a separate chapter)! Research shows that nucleotides in breastmilk increase at night. This might indicate the role that nucleotides play in sleep homeostasis and the relaxing effect it has on the baby.[2] Simply put, your milk is putting your baby to sleep! This is what is supposed to happen; your baby is meant to fall asleep at your breast. This is normal and beautiful. There are always exceptions to this: there are babies who fall asleep happily on their own. However, for most babies, falling asleep while breastfeeding is the biological norm.

2. Sánchez, C, et al. The possible role of human milk nucleotides as sleep inducers. *Nutritional Neuroscience.* 2009; 12: 2–8.

You can see why people make millions of dollars selling sleep-training books; books filled with step-by-step instructions on how to get babies to fall asleep and stay asleep on their own. The process is simply not supposed to happen this way! Most babies communicate the only way they can—through tears—that they just need to be cuddled. Touch through breastfeeding, cuddling, carrying, holding: this is what our little ones need.

If you have a baby who happily falls asleep without breastfeeding or cuddles, awesome! Go with it! While this is not the experience of most breastfeeding mothers, there are definitely cases where this happens and no, there is not something wrong with your baby. You just happened to have a little munchkin who is easily settled. If they are happy to be put down awake and fall asleep on their own then definitely work with that and see if you can encourage your baby to continue this. I mean, why not?! Follow the lead of your baby and what is working for them.

All of the pictures shown in this section are of my youngest boy after he had fallen asleep at the breast. How could anyone argue with that little face? He was happy, content, and full. He ate, fell asleep, and then I would put him down (or cuddle him) for his nap or for the night (Haha! By "night" I mean for an hour or two until he woke again to breastfeed)!

Some people argue that babies need to learn how to fall asleep alone (without cuddles or breastfeeds). Some people claim that their children will always need to be comforted to sleep if we create perceived bad habits by feeding or cuddling them to sleep. Why is this? All three of my babies have been breastfed to sleep. My eldest boy now barely kisses me goodnight before he reads a book and then falls asleep all by himself. My middle boy, who is 8, gets a book read to him and then he falls asleep all by himself. My youngest has gone from breastfeeding to sleep pretty much every night, to being rocked to sleep by my husband, to falling asleep in his own bed all alone with the door closed…because he likes it that way! He will now occasionally fall asleep while breastfeeding, it's about being flexible. All three of my children fall asleep on their own, all without sleep training of any sort. Yay for gentle parenting and mothering through breastfeeding!

There are three VERY IMPORTANT secrets to parenting…

1. TRUST YOUR INSTINCTS.

2. TRUST YOUR INSTINCTS.

3. TRUST YOUR INSTINCTS.

If people are giving you well-meaning advice to let your baby learn to fall asleep alone (in other words, CRY) and it doesn't feel right to you then TRUST YOUR INSTINCTS and breastfeed. Smile at these people and ignore them. There will come a time when your little one no longer breastfeeds to sleep. Then you will miss these quiet, beautiful breastfeeding moments. Especially when your tween is yelling out, "I hate you! I hate this house! I'm moving out!" Then you will REALLY miss those moments.

FEELING
OVERWHELMED?
CANCEL YOUR
PLANS...
GET INTO BED
WITH YOUR
BABY... AND
CHILL OUT
FOR A BIT.

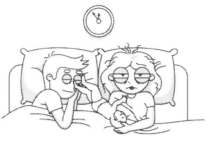

Am I Creating Bad Habits?

Time to Relax and Find your Inner Marsupial…

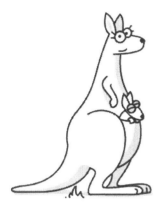

I cannot tell you how many times I have been contacted by someone asking if they are "creating bad habits" by breastfeeding their child to sleep, bedsharing, co-sleeping or breastfeeding through the night and on demand. Often times this is never something the mother has just thought of on her own at 2am, but a comment here or there from a well-meaning mother, grandmother, aunt or friend who suggests that they are creating a bad habit by doing these things. Then the mother goes into a tailspin of questioning what she is doing wrong and heads online to find baby sleep books which reinforce this idea of spoiling.

The definition of "bad habit" as defined by The Dictionary of Modern Medicine is, "A patterned behaviour regarded as detrimental to one's physical or mental health, which is often linked to a lack of self-control."[1] Could you imagine describing breastfeeding to sleep or throughout the night as being detrimental to your child's physical or mental health? Both waking at night

---

1. "Bad Habit." Segen's Medical Dictionary. 2001. Farlex, Inc. http://medical-dictionary.thefreedictionary.com/Bad+Habit Published 2001. Accessed November 2, 2014.

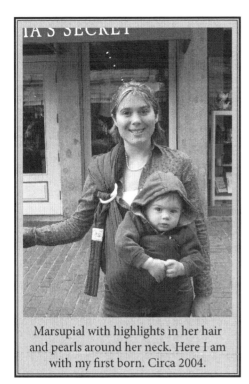

Marsupial with highlights in her hair and pearls around her neck. Here I am with my first born. Circa 2004.

and falling asleep while breastfeeding are the biological norms. This is not only true for newborns, but for many toddlers as well. What we really need is a pouch like a kangaroo to fit our tiny little helpless newborns (and growing toddlers) in.

Since our babies are born so prematurely compared to other mammals, it is important (and actually imperative) to frequently hold, and breastfeed them. Breastfeeding your baby to sleep is the easiest, most natural thing in the world. Most babies do not fall asleep easily without a cuddle and/or a breastfeed. This is not creating a bad habit; it is what happens naturally. Looking at the face of a child who has fallen asleep at the breast will tell you how normal and awesome it is. We are bringing comfort and security to our babies by doing what is most natural. By creating this safe place through cuddles and breastfeeds, we are then, in turn, creating children who feel secure enough in themselves to be confident and independent in the future. Just like the marsupial kangaroo joey that jumps in and out of the pouch to explore the world around him, so do our growing children. This comfort at the breast continues as they grow into toddlerhood.

Humans are altiricial which means they require nourishment. "Altricial" comes from the latin word *alere* which means to nurse, to rear or to nourish.[2] Humans require attention and round the clock care for an extended period of time following their birth.

2.Ehrlich, Paul. *The Birder's Handbook.* New York: Simon & Schuster; 1988

For humans, it is even longer than other mammals. We are really much more like marsupials than mammals! Where is my pouch?!

Marsupials birth their babies much sooner than humans which requires their little ones to stay in the pouch to survive. Although human babies do not need a pouch for survival, they are born so much earlier (developmentally wise) compared to other many other mammals which is why our babies require so much more attention. There has been an estimation that a human fetus would have to undergo a gestation period of 18 to 21 months instead of the usual nine to be born at a neurological and cognitive development stage comparable to that of a chimpanzee newborn.[3] Our babies survival does depend on our constant attention 24/7 which would be made so much easier if we had a pouch to put them in!

Marsupials are an infraclass of mammals. While they are similar, the fact that they have their awesome and amazing pouch makes it so much easier for them. Actually, the baby finds the pouch and the nipple themselves! As unique as this sounds, human babies are capable of finding the nipple and latching independently as well. There are many videos online which show the awesomeness of baby self-attachment.

Would you ever think to tell the mother kangaroo that she needs to de-latch her little baby from the nipple and that she really should not be breastfeeding her baby so often? Would you think to ask her if her baby is a "good" baby and sleeping "through the night"? Would you think to suggest to this kangaroo mother that she puts her baby down because she is spoiling it? No! Of course not! Why are we seen as so different then? We have babies who are born very prematurely compared to other mammals. We have babies who require frequent breastfeeds (on demand) and comfort 24/7. And we have babies who are just not content without us or the boob. We are much more similar to marsupials

3. Wong, Kate. Why Humans Give Birth to Helpless Babies. *Scientific America.* http://blogs.scientificamerican.com/observations/2012/08/28/why-humans-give-birth-to-helpless-babies/ Published August 28, 2012. Accessed January 22, 2015.

than we realize…we just have to buy our pouch because we're not born with one.

By finding your inner marsupial you can take away so much of the stress and questioning of the early weeks and months of motherhood. The kangaroo mother does not think twice about having her baby (and growing toddler joey) nursing all the time. If you were out living on a mountain having never heard of self-settling, schedules or creating bad habits would you even think to do anything BUT keep your baby or toddler close and breastfeed them frequently?

You cannot breastfeed your child too frequently. You cannot hold your child too often. You cannot create bad habits by feeding on demand, to sleep, or throughout the night. Doing these things is biologically normal…and important. Find your inner marsupial and put your feet up. You can relax knowing you are meeting the needs of your child in the most natural way possible… as nature intended.

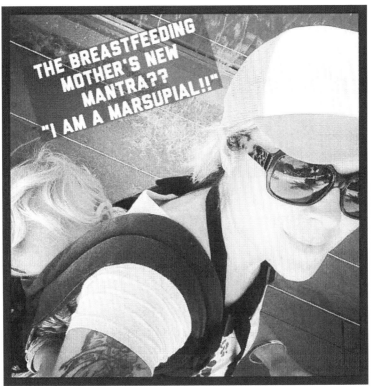

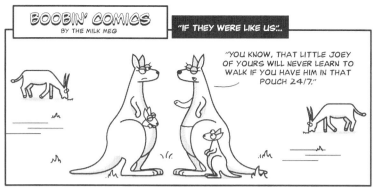

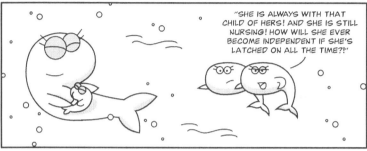

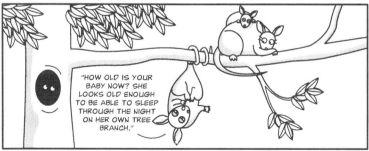

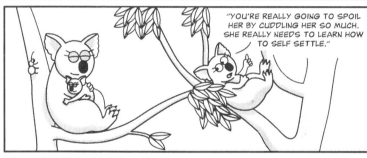

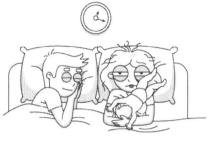

Tandem Breastfeeding and Bedsharing

Tandem breastfeeding is when a mother is feeding both her baby and her older child at the same time. Sometimes a woman will be feeding her two oldest while pregnant with her third! Women are amazing!

Many women who are pregnant while breastfeeding get a bit anxious when thinking about the new baby arriving and how it is all going to work! They have questions about HOW it's actually going to happen. Who do I feed first? Will my toddler start breastfeeding as frequently as my newborn? Will I have enough milk? Every woman will experience different things. Some will see a decrease in their milk supply, some will feel an extreme aversion to breastfeeding and others will have no issues at all! Their milk will continue to keep up with supply as normal, throughout their entire pregnancy and they will not mind breastfeeding while pregnant. It's really an individual experience. There is no research to show that breastfeeding during a normal pregnancy is harmful for you or your unborn baby,[1] however if you have questions, it's important to seek advice from a health care professional who is breastfeeding-friendly and will give you evidence-based information. There are actually no specific medical guidelines that exist to define a situation where it may be risky to continue breastfeeding while pregnant.[1] Breastfeeding

---

1. La Leche League International: pregnancy and tandem nursing. In: *The Breastfeeding Answer Book.* 3rd ed. Schaumburg, Illinois: La Leche League International; 2003: 405-410.

causes contractions with the uterus, however this happens naturally throughout your pregnancy (whether you feel it or not!), including when you have sex.

Parents also have many questions about sleep. If you are bedsharing or co-sleeping with your firstborn, then chances are you are thinking about doing the same with your newborn. Some women find it easier to night-wean and slowly transition their firstborn out of the bed and into another bed before the new baby arrives. Other women will continue to bedshare with their baby and toddler. Both options are possible and you can continue to follow the safe co-sleeping guidelines while doing this. It is important to make sure your baby is not next to your toddler. You can put a couple of mattresses together so you can put your toddler on his own or you can get a larger bed. King size beds make great family beds!

Here is Jade's story about night-time mothering through breastfeeding, while tandem feeding her toddler and baby!

"When I had my first baby, breastfeeding came pretty naturally for me. I love the bonding and the nurturing feeling I get when I am breastfeeding. Although we had bought a cot and a bassinet, it seemed more natural for my husband and I to bedshare with our new baby, so we went with what felt right.

My daughter was 7 months old when I became pregnant with my son. She breastfed throughout my entire pregnancy and I remember her saying "Mama your milk tastes funny." She still continued anyway though! When my son was born, we struggled to breastfeed properly for the first few weeks, but he was feeding like a pro before too long. At this stage my daughter was 16 months old and still fed regularly, even throughout the night, so she was pretty happy when my milk changed again. I remember spending heaps of time on the couch tandem breastfeeding my babies. Their bond was incredible and they would often hold hands while they were feeding. We still continued to bedshare which made it easier to feed two children throughout the night and, needless to say, we got a king size bed. There

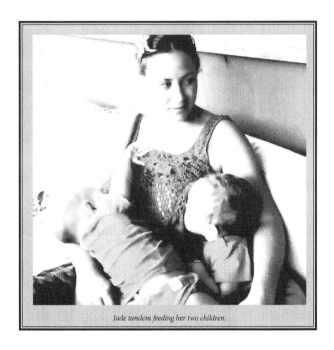

Jade tandem feeding her two children.

were times that I struggled, but mostly it was an amazing experience to tandem breastfeed and I think my children still share a very special bond together.

When it came to night-weaning my daughter, she got upset at first but if she was too upset, I would let her breastfeed and try again the next day. She eventually just stopped asking when she woke up throughout the night. Instead of breastfeeding her for comfort she would ask for cuddles to go back to sleep. She began to be quite proud of herself and say, 'I can have sushabush (her name for breastfeeding) now because the sun is up.' I would still breastfeed her to get to sleep at night though and when she woke up in the night she would look out the window and say. 'No sushabush because the sun is not up.' I used the exact approach with my son. He seemed to respond in the very same way. He sometimes cried but would always find comfort in cuddles. In the beginning if he was too upset, I would let him breastfeed. I would also feed them throughout the night if they were sick or had a fever because I found it more difficult to soothe them with just cuddles if they were unwell.

I found it so much easier to breastfeed my babies to sleep rather than letting them self-settle. I never liked hearing either of them cry, even for a short time, so I would pick them up straight away if they were upset. It just felt right to me and natural. Without even really thinking about it I would generally always comfort them through breastfeeding. It seemed the easiest and most natural way to get them to sleep."

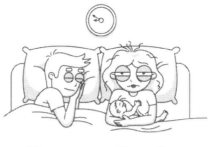

Reverse Cycling

Goodbye day boob, hello night boob.

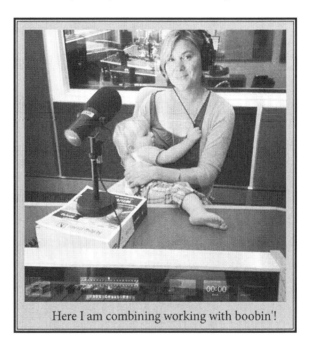

Here I am combining working with boobin'!

Many mothers find that as their babies grow, they will start to "reverse cycle" with their usual breastfeeding routine. I remember with my first boy thinking what a weirdo he was! He was not only continuing to breastfeed happily beyond babyhood (which for me as a first time mum was a whole new thing) but he was starting to breastfeed less during the day and more at night! It was not something I was expecting and had not read anything about this. Of course I immediately started to wonder what was wrong and if it was something I was doing since blaming ourselves is a common past time of us mothers.

Reverse cycling just means that instead of their usual night waking they will start to wake a bit more frequently to make up for the boobin' time that they missed out on during the day. This does not only happen to mothers who return to work but will also happen when your child starts to notice the world around them. Instead of breastfeeding happily they will pop off frequently, look around to see what interesting things are happening and then want to get off of your lap before they have even had a decent breastfeed. No worries at all for them though as they will make up for all those missed session at night!

Returning to work as a breastfeeding mother can be very anxiety producing! We have so many questions; will our babies be happy without us there, if we will be able to pump enough milk while separated and of course…how will we continue to get enough sleep, breastfeed during the night as we always have AND actually continue to function as a working adult? Many of the breastfeeding mothers I have spoken to who work outside the home are really thankful for all of the night time cuddles and breastfeeds.

While some mothers do decide to night-wean, many others continue to co-sleep or bedshare while breastfeeding their little ones. This can help keep up your milk supply as the more you breastfeed your child when you are with them, the easier it will be for you to keep up your supply when you return to work or start to have more prolonged times apart from your child. Pumping during those missed breastfeeding sessions is of course crucial to your supply, but what you do when you are actually WITH your baby is just as important. Night time breastfeeding can be a great way to help with this.

Here is Rebecca's experience with keeping up her supply and breastfeeding at night after returning to work:

> "After my son was born I stayed home with him for 3 months. I went back to work 2 days a week (10 hour days). I would pump every 2 1/2

to 3 hours at first. I work at a veterinary clinic so I would just use an empty exam room. He is now 10 1/2 months old. We still bed share and breastfeed on demand when I am with him. I now pump every 4 hours at work. On days that I work I notice he wakes more at night to breastfeed. He wakes on average 3 to 6 times a night. It is nice to have him right next to me to roll over and nurse him and go right back to sleep. My little man loves his booby."

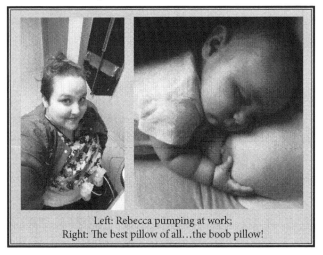

Left: Rebecca pumping at work;
Right: The best pillow of all…the boob pillow!

Tamara (who has lived in different countries around Asia) had this to share about her breastfeeding, sleep and work experiences with her son who was ill:

"Throughout Asia, maternity leave is for 70 consecutive days including weekends and holidays. My son came to work with me and stayed in a room at work with his carer. During breaks I would go to him to feed. My son became ill at 6 months due to pollution in China and stopped taking in any nourishment aside from breast milk from age 7-18 or so months. He refused bottles and I am pretty useless at pumping so we needed to be together to keep him alive. He breastfed every 3 hours until he was well over 18 months which was when we moved to Bangkok. Due to his illness, bed sharing was our only option if any of us were to sleep, plus, by lying on my chest I could monitor his breathing and keep him elevated. At my current workplace we fought for three years to get a mother's room, which is finally in place now. Prior to that teachers feed in their classrooms (which is what I did when my son was young)."

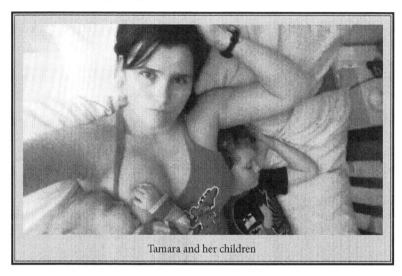

Tamara and her children

Meeting your child's night time needs through breastfeeding can be incredibly helpful during an illness. Breastfeeding can help clear your child's nose, calm a coughing spell and help them sleep.

Joanne feels as though the night time bedsharing and breastfeeding helps them to reconnect after the day apart:

"I went back to work when my little guy was one. I work full time and was stressed about how it would all work but neither of us were ready to wean. Everyone around me told me to wean him and put him on formula or cow's milk in a bottle when I came back to work. There were many occasions when I sat in tears just not feeling right about that. I just decided to keep breastfeeding and see what happened.

Prior to returning to work James was breastfeeding a lot still but as soon as I started leaving him each day that increased. Now he is attached to me from the minute he wakes up and especially when I get home in the afternoon.

On weekends and when I'm not working he breastfeeds all through the day.

From birth he mainly slept in his cot but was slowly making his way into our bed. After I returned to work I brought him into our bed where he now still permanently sleeps. I missed him each day and love that time at night where he's still, quiet and we thoroughly enjoy the cuddles. He breastfeeds all through the night – sometimes more than others. I feel bed sharing and breastfeeding help us to reconnect."

Not every mother will find that bedsharing or co-sleeping is the answer for them after they return to work. Maybe you find that your child sleeps worse when they are with you or maybe you do not get as much sleep. Listen to your instincts and do what feels right for you and your little night time booby lover.

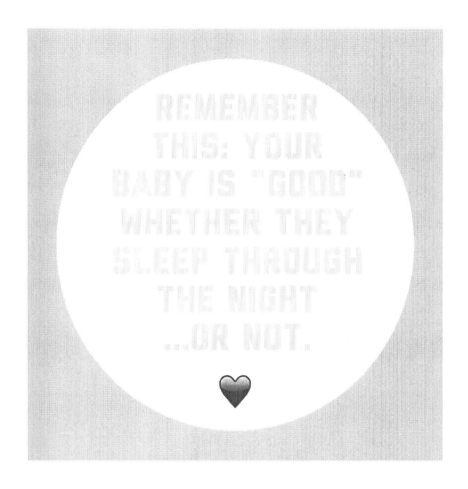

REMEMBER THIS: YOUR BABY IS "GOOD" WHETHER THEY SLEEP THROUGH THE NIGHT ...OR NOT.

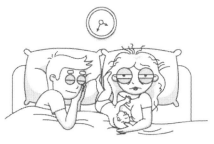

How Much Sleep Does My Child Need?

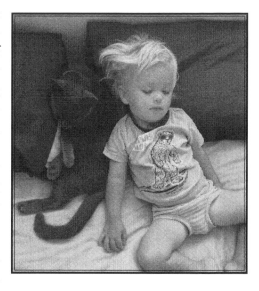

Sleep becomes a bit of an obsession when we have our babies. Even if we are happy with how our baby is sleeping (or not sleeping), we are constantly asked if our baby is GOOD. Is she sleeping? How long is she sleeping for? Are you getting any sleep? How much is she napping? We think about it, worry about it, and generally experience some sort of anxiety about it throughout the early years of parenthood. So, what's the deal with sleep deprivation? Will my child be doomed if they do not sleep enough?!

Ok, so there is no question that sleep is important, BUT people are missing the big picture here. So often I hear people go ON AND ON about how important and crucial it is for your baby or toddler to be getting ENOUGH sleep. Yes, lack of sleep can cause all sorts of problems, but how do you know when it has gone from normal to problem?

Let's start with normal sleep behavior of a breastfed baby…

1.   Babies will often fall asleep happily at the breast, but will wake if put down and therefore have shorter naps if they are not held or put back to sleep by breastfeeding.

2.   Babies will often wake up about 30–45 minutes after falling asleep for their nap during the lighter part of the sleep cycle.

3.   Babies and toddlers will wake frequently to breastfeed at night.

4.   Babies and toddlers tend to cluster feed in the pre-dawn hours leading up to the eventual time-to-wake-up boob.

5.   Babies will go through cycles. For some weeks or months, they might nap quite well. Then they will start to nap for a shorter time period and need more frequent breastfeeds during the nap to stay asleep. You might describe them as unsettled or cranky. This could go on for a few days or weeks. You will start to go insane… and then magically they will start to sleep longer for their naps and be more settled at night. You may, or may not, find the reason why this happened.

6.   Sometimes a baby's nap will happen while breastfeeding. They will happily latch on and NOT LET GO for the entire nap… this is what I like to call "the nap boob." This can happen sometimes and will often be random, possibly due to baby's increased need for cuddling, or if fighting an illness or feeling unsettled for a number of reasons.

7.   Each of your children may be completely different with their sleep patterns, even if you breastfeed them and mother them the same exact way! My middle boy LOVED and still LOVES to sleep! He happily fell asleep while breastfeeding until he was three and a half years old and breastfed for a nap every single day until he weaned. He would not only nap for at least two hours, but would also easily fall asleep at the breast at night at 7:30pm. No problems at all… and seriously, the kid still loves his sleep!

THIS IS ALL NORMAL! THERE IS NO PROBLEM HERE PEOPLE! THESE SLEEP PATTERNS ARE COMPLETELY NORMAL FOR BREASTFED BABIES AND TODDLERS!

When will I know it's time for my toddler to stop napping? Here are some signs:

1. Baby will stop breastfeeding to sleep (and not just as a phase, but for quite a while) and you have to get creative!

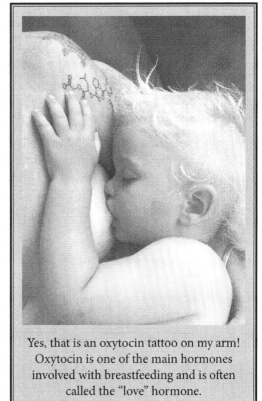

Yes, that is an oxytocin tattoo on my arm! Oxytocin is one of the main hormones involved with breastfeeding and is often called the "love" hormone.

With my youngest boy it started to get ridiculous! He stopped breastfeeding to sleep for his nap, so I would use the baby carrier. Then when that stopped working, I would put him in the carrier while vacuuming! My house was ridiculously clean every day, but eventually the vacuum stopped working too. It's great to figure out little tricks (and my tricks gave me an extra six months of naps!), but eventually they will stop working.

2. Baby will nap but it will take you FOREVER to get them to fall asleep.

3. Baby will start to show signs of being able to make it through the afternoon without having a meltdown! They will make it to 6:30pm (or whatever time you are happy with putting them to bed) and will easily fall asleep at the breast or while being cuddled.

4. Baby will start going to bed REALLY late if there is a mid-day nap. The baby will nap later in the afternoon (when you finally get the child to sleep!) but will then torture you into the late hours of the night while you hold your eyelids open with toothpicks.

Literally days before I was going to send my final book edit off to the printer, a new research article was published by *JAMA Pediatrics*.[1] They interviewed parents during pregnancy, when their child reached 18 months, and then again at 5 years old. Questions were asked about how frequently their child woke and if their child had any behavioral or emotional problems.

The study concluded that, "Toddlers who slept less than ten hours a night or woke frequently at night tended to have more emotional and behavioral problems at age 5." Sounds scary, huh?! This is the sort of research that sleep trainers/sleep consultants/ baby whisperers will quote to parents to support their methods of cry-it-out, doing the "pick-up, put-down" method of sleep training or "shooshing" babies to sleep without touching them or cuddling them. Let me bring up a few points about this though...

1. This study includes NOTHING about whether these parents slept with or without their toddlers at 18 months. Why is this important? Because if your 18 month old is sleeping with you or next to you in the bed, chances are they sleep happily next to you and they stir (but not actually fully wake up) to breastfeed a few times. Breastfed children at 18 months usually wake to breastfeed a few times. This is NOT a "sleep problem," this is the biological norm. This is what children do when they are breastfed and bedshare. This has been happening FOREVER. Why would something that is historically the norm then lead to emotionally and behaviorally troubled children? This makes absolutely NO sense from an anthropological perspective.

---

1. Borge, S, et al. Later emotional and behavioral problems associated with sleep problems in toddlers. *JAMA Pediatrics*. doi:10.1001/ jamapediatrics.2015.0187. Published April 13, 2015. Accessed April 16, 2015.

2. This study has no data that shows if the child is breastfed, formula fed or mixed fed. This is important as well, as frequent night-waking to breastfeed (as mentioned above) is usually related to a child sleeping with their mother some or all of the time, which leads to more frequent stirring... but again for many of us, not actually waking up distressed.

3. This study did not address HOW the parents responded to their child. Did they cuddle them? Bring them into their bed? Did the child actually fall asleep next to their parents or in their own bed? Babies and toddlers who sleep with or very close to their parents are often barely waking, as they are immediately put onto the boob or comforted back to sleep.

This. Is. Normal.

This study does not take into account that frequent night-waking to breastfeed with bedsharing and co-sleeping toddlers is the biological norm; this is what we have done as a human race around the world in every society until just recent history, when some people decided that babies and toddlers should sleep ten hours straight.

Do not be scared into sleep training. MOTHERING THROUGH BREASTFEEDING AT NIGHT IS THE BIOLOGICAL NORM. Not a "problem."

Is sleep important? Of course, but scaring parents into sleep training by quoting these research articles is harmful and unfair to exhausted parents. Sleep For Kids[2] website states the following for sleep guidelines:

Age	Total Sleep (hours)
0-2 months	10.5-18
2-12 months	14-15
1-3 years	12-14
3-5 years	11-13
5-12 years	10-11

Web MD's guide to sleep[3] states:

Age	Total Sleep (hours)
4 weeks	15-16
1-4 months	14-15
4-12 months	14-15
1-3 years	12-14

---

2. Children and Sleep. http://www.sleepforkids.org/html/sheet.html Accessed February 12, 2015.

3. How Much Sleep Do Children Need? http://www.webmd.com/parenting/guide/sleep-children Published February 28, 2014. Accessed February 12, 2015.

The National Sleep Foundation[4] has a much more general approach to their recommendation:

Age	Total Sleep (hours)
Newborn	14-17
Infants	12-15
Toddlers	11-14
Preschoolers	10-13
School-aged children	9-11

Notice something? They are not identical! There are variations in many of the sleep charts (it's not an exact science!).

So what is the bottom line? Look at the WHOLE PICTURE.

As concluded by the research from the National Sleep Foundation,[3] sufficient sleep duration requirements vary throughout our lives and from person to person. The researchers stated that the recommendations given in the article were guidelines for healthy individuals. Guidelines are not black and white. There will always be differences between children, even within your own family and regardless of whether you breastfed them to sleep, had hard-core routines, or were a bit relaxed about the whole thing.

Look at your child. Look at how she is responding to the changes in her sleep patterns. Does she need more sleep and struggle if she misses her nap? Then get creative… breastfeed her to sleep in a carrier, go out in the morning so she falls asleep on the ride or walk home, vacuum like me, get into bed with her and take a nap together while breastfeeding on and off… whatever it takes! Drop the nap completely when that stops working as well.

---

4. Hirshkowitz M, et al, National Sleep Foundation's sleep time duration recommendations: methodology and results summary. *Sleep Health* (2015), http://dx.doi.org/10.1016/j.sleh.2014.12.010

When I realized my youngest was giving up his nap, I cried! I was not ready! He was only two and I felt the pressure to have him nap still! But once I let the idea of the nap go we were both happier. I stopped spending so much time trying to put him to sleep and we just enjoyed the day together. Plus, I really enjoyed his new early bed time. Is your child meeting his developmental milestones? Is he happy and healthy? Great!

Trust your instincts and follow the lead of your child. Then keep on boobin'!

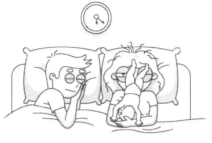

How to Get More Sleep

Without Doing Cry-It-Out

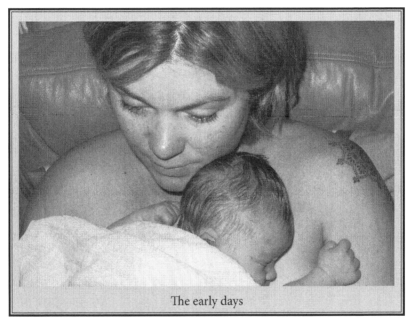

The early days

Let's focus on US! Not our babies…

Remember what it was like way back in the day when it was awesome and exciting to stay up all night? After having a baby our attitude about late nights changes just a bit. As new mums we can feel so overwhelmed and we are bombarded with various advice (usually about sleep and breastfeeding), much of which has us going against our motherly instincts. But what if we were able to change the way we think about babies and sleep? Instead of focusing on the negative (the why... why... why questions focused on our baby) focus on the positive and yourself, focus on what you CAN change! From reading my book, you know it is completely normal for babies and toddlers, who are breastfed on demand, to wake frequently and breastfeed. I am actually surprised if I come across a woman who has a baby or toddler who sleeps well at night. Instead of partying all night we are breastfeeding all night. This is motherhood.

Try asking yourself these questions:

What can I do to get more sleep? Who is available to come over for a couple of hours to help me today? What can I leave until tomorrow? What can I reschedule today so I don't have to leave the house?

Yes, you can train your baby to sleep longer and sleep by themselves if you leave them to cry and practice sleep training, responsive settling, or the cry-it-out method. Call it what you will but it all equals the same thing—your baby is in distress and not getting his needs met. A baby crying is a baby communicating. Research[1] shows just how stressful it is for babies who are left to cry. Their stress hormone levels are raised even after they stop crying. Thankfully there is another answer! We focus so much on our babies sleeping that we lose sight of the things that we are capable of changing—things that will help us feel less tired and give us increased energy throughout the day and night.

As a mum to three breastfed boys, I understand extreme tiredness! I would GET CRANKY AND EXHAUSTED! I would complain to my husband! I would cry! I felt as though I might go insane from lack of sleep at times! Yet most of the time just changing my thought patterns and HOW I thought about the situation could really change my feelings about it. We are so focused on the night that we forget all of the things we might be able to do during the day. Try this on for size...

---

1. Middlemiss W, Granger D, Goldberg W, Nathans L. Asynchrony of mother–infant hypothalamic–pituitary–adrenal axis activity following extinction of infant crying responses induced during the transition to sleep. *Early Human Development.* 2012; 88, 227–232.

1. Instead of: "Why won't my baby sleep?" Try: "What can I do to get more sleep?"

You are going to get cranky at me for saying this but I'm saying it anyway! SLEEP WHEN YOUR BABY SLEEPS DURING THE DAY!!!! Do not do laundry or cleaning or TV watching or Facebook checking (unless it is my page of course). SLEEP. So simple but SO VERY IMPORTANT.

People get really upset at me sometimes when I post this on my Facebook page. I think for many of us, the last thing we think we can do is sleep. I'm not talking about a three hour nap here though. I'm just saying it's important to STOP what you are doing for a few minutes. Even if you cannot fall asleep, just lie there with your eyes closed. You do not have to be sleeping to be resting.

Hire someone to come during the day so you can get twenty minutes of shut eye. Put an ad in your local newspaper and find a babysitter in training or mother's helper who loves babies and will charge next to nothing to just hold your baby or play with your toddler or older children while you take a short nap or lie down.

Go to bed when your baby goes to bed. This might mean putting older children to bed earlier as well. Put them to bed early or with a book if they can read and everyone goes to sleep. Have a big sleeping party together on the floor if you need to.

From boobin' mum Sarah:

> "I just go to bed when my baby goes to bed! Yes it does mean that I'm missing out on some quiet time after he falls asleep but it can really help when I need some extra rest."

2. Instead of: " Why is my baby waking so much?" Try: "Who is available to come over for a couple of hours to help me today?"

It is normal for babies and toddlers to have nights where they wake frequently. This could be due to teething, going through a developmental milestone, growth spurt, general crankiness, getting sick, etc. When your baby has a night like this then see if you can find a family member, friend, or hire a mother's helper to come over. If you can afford it, hire someone to come in and clean once a week or every two weeks.

Find a mother friend who is happy to alternate time between your houses. While they are watching your baby and/or children you can rest. Then the next time you go over to her house and do the same when she is tired.

3. Instead of: "Will I ALWAYS have to breastfeed him to sleep?" Try: "What am I wanting to do that is making me feel this is a chore or burden?"

If I was annoyed that I had to breastfeed my baby to sleep at night it is almost always because there was something I would have rather been doing. Cleaning the kitchen, watching a movie with my husband, reading to my other children, or just doing nothing! Ha! What a crazy idea! If I changed my thinking though, then I could appreciate the needs of my baby at that time and stop being so obsessed with what it was that I had to do at that moment. The kitchen could wait, I could fall asleep next to my husband on the couch if I had to (at least we would be together!) and I could read to my children tomorrow.

4. Instead of: "How can I get my baby to sleep longer?" Try: "What can I leave until tomorrow?"

It is completely normal for babies to take short naps sometimes and only want to be held while sleeping. You might want to invest in a comfortable baby carrier that you can carry your baby in while they sleep. Although this will not be ideal every day for you, there will be days where this is your magical answer. I was able to get many things done around the house this way and even as he grew into toddlerhood I was still able to carry him around comfortably on my back. I could also sit down and work at the computer with him on my back.

Let go of the Ultimate Mother thing. We all have to let some stuff go when we are tired. The house might get a bit messy, your legs might not get shaved for a month, and you might have to eat your lunch standing for two weeks in a row… but it does get easier! I promise.

You cannot do it all, all at once. You cannot bake paleo muffins, make homemade soap, and construct a DIY bookshelf you found on Pinterest all within the same day. IT CAN WAIT UNTIL YOU ARE LESS SLEEP-DEPRIVED! And think: easy dinners! This will save your sanity too.

GET SUPPORT, WAIT AS LONG AS POSSIBLE BEFORE RETURNING TO WORK, AND FIND THE SLEEPING ARRANGEMENT THAT WORKS FOR YOU TO GET MORE SLEEP—WHETHER IT'S CO-SLEEPING, BEDSHARING, OR YOUR BABY SLEEPING IN HER OWN ROOM. We are all in this together. Let's support each other! It's all about building community support.

*Most important: Ask for help when you need it! Especially if you feel as though you are feeling so overwhelmed that you cannot care for your baby or you are feeling depressed.

Alternatives to Cry-It-Out

Because every baby is just asking for a cuddle!

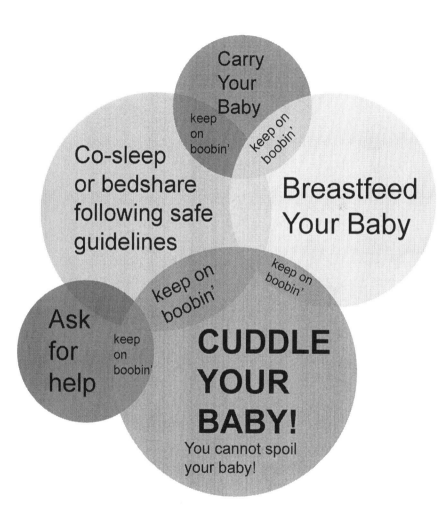

Carry Your Baby

keep on boobin'

keep on boobin'

Co-sleep or bedshare following safe guidelines

Breastfeed Your Baby

keep on boobin'

keep on boobin'

Ask for help

keep on boobin'

CUDDLE YOUR BABY!
You cannot spoil your baby!

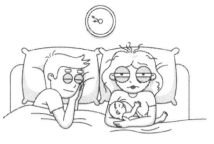

I'm a Gentle Parent...
But I'm Losing my Shit

I'd like to take a break in the middle of my sleep book to address something that I think is not addressed enough. Sometimes as a mother you are going to completely lose your shit. Yup, it's true. You will consider yourself a gentle parent and be conscious of being patient and accepting your nocturnal child for who she is. Then it will all come crumbling down. Maybe you are experiencing pure and utter exhaustion right now, similar to the time I was trying so hard to put my youngest to bed (without luck) that I just lost it. I yelled. I cried. I took him out of the baby carrier, ran out to the living room and announced to my husband, "I can't flippin' do this anymore! I am exhausted! He won't go to bed! I'm done! I'm done!" OK maybe that's happened more than once…

You see, gentle parenting does not mean that we are walking around in a hypnotic, meditative state thanking the universe for giving us this amazing, high-spirited, sleepless child. No. It can mean that we lose it. It can mean that we get sick of carrying our babies around. We get really tired when breastfeeding for hours some nights, while our baby is wide awake looking up at us as if to say, "What? I'm awake and that's it. Just accept it." Some days, some nights… it's really hard. The main problem with how so many of us live today is that we are alone. If we are lucky we have a partner or family member we live with who can help us, but even with another person or two, we are sometimes so lonely. We wake at 2am and feel as though we are the only person awake in the world. We sit and cry all alone because we feel as though we cannot possibly function on such little sleep. We start to feel as though maybe we are going crazy. We think surely we are doing something wrong? It's all because I'm an attachment parent! It's all my fault!

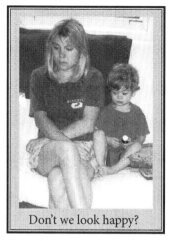

Don't we look happy?

OK. Here's the thing… no matter what type of parenting style you follow, there will be moments when you feel guilty. Moments where you cry and cry questioning what you have done or how you should have done it differently. Should I have put her in the cot straight away? Should I have co-slept instead of putting her in the cot? Should I have stopped boobin' her to sleep? Should I have stopped putting her in her cot to self-settle? Should I have gotten her used to the bouncy seat instead of being in the baby carrier? The thing to remember though is that one day you will look back and reflect on all of this. One day you will think about all of these little bumps in the parenting road. If during this time you can trust your own instincts and follow the lead of your child then you will know that you chose the right path for you and your family.

Listen to your little ones. They will let you know if what you are doing is working for them or not. Seek help when you need it and remember we are all in this together. There are millions of us awake at 2 am breastfeeding our babies. We are all losing our shit at various times, in varying degrees of severity. Remember that breastfeeding is a relationship, it is not just about our children. If I am feeling mother burnout it's usually because I'm giving 110% to my children and forgetting all about myself! That is not a good lesson to teach my kids and it can also be a direct path to losing it. Seek support! We cannot do this on our own.

If at any time you feel unable to care for yourself or your baby please seek help from a health care professional. Postpartum depression, or the baby blues, does not always show itself as sadness, but can be experienced as sensations of feeling overwhelmed or numb.

EVEN GENTLE PARENTS LOSE THEIR SHIT. SEEK SUPPORT. TRUST YOUR INSTINCTS. KEEP ON BOOBIN'

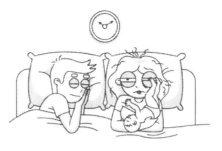

Routines and Demand Feeding

…can you have both?

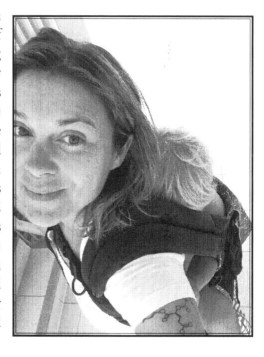

There is a common misconception that if you are breastfeeding on demand (by following baby's cues instead of the clock) then you cannot have routines. This could not be further from the truth. Babies and children LOVE routines (or rituals as I like to call them) and combining both free range boobin' and rituals can make for very happy babies and very happy mothers.

So why even bother if we are boobin' all the time randomly? Because routines can really help your baby to understand what is happening! If you start these rituals with them, then you create cues, so they start to understand that it's time to sleep. For some babies, these rituals can be helpful. Do not mistakenly think that these are the magical answers for getting your baby to fall asleep on the boob instantly… and then sleep for three hours straight! Yes, maybe this will happen for you! But remember that this is another tool in your boobin' toolbox that can help. Of course it is also important to realize that every baby is an individual. Follow their lead and do what works for them (and for you).

I must admit, as first time parents, my husband and I loved it when our baby was really little so we could continue to go out and do most everything we did before—we just happened to have a baby with us! However as he got a bit older it became clear that he was starting to fall into patterns on his own (around his nap and bed time) and we knew that our care-free days of coming and going as we pleased needed to change a bit so we could take into account his natural body rhythms. Even if you do nothing around rituals or routines your baby will eventually find their own anyway. Don't stress too much about this in the early weeks. This is a time to adjust to motherhood and relax as much as you can with your little one.

You can begin these routines right from the start though if you think they will be helpful for you! Whenever you feel you want to try incorporating these then please do! There is no age that is too early or too late. Go with what your own instincts and your baby are telling you. Our little guy made it very clear to us when this change needed to happen.

Ideas for rituals around nap time

There are a few different ways you can incorporate routines around nap times.

- **Breastfeed!** This is always my first suggestion. If your baby falls asleep while breastfeeding then try this first.
- **Baby wearing.** Get a baby carrier and wear your baby. There are a variety of different ones but try to find one that you can easily breastfeed in. This way you can combine both baby wearing and breastfeeding at the same time if needed.
- **Swaddling.** This might help your little baby if you are not going to hold or lie with her during the nap but are putting her down on her own, after falling asleep.

- **Sing.** My mother-in-law always jokes about how the song she used to sing to my husband to put him to sleep was the stupidest little song and how she cannot sing! Your baby will not care though. The repetition of singing the same song can be very soothing.

- **Drive or take your baby for a walk.** With my second-born, I had my day organized so I knew I'd always be driving home from somewhere (if I had to go out) or walking back from somewhere with him in the pram (stroller) at the same time every day. This is my child who LOVED and still loves to sleep. He would fall asleep every single day really easily, either in the car, on the way home in the pram, or on the boob. I'd just make sure I did one of these things at the same time, every day, around when his nap time was.

Ideas for rituals around bed time

- **Bath.** OK I must tell you something here though. So many books and articles suggest bathing your baby or toddler (or child) as the start to a bedtime routine. THIS NEVER WORKED FOR ME! Baths completely hype my children up! They would get out of the bath and then run around like wild maniacs for half an hour. I'm not sure if this actually works for some people but it must because I read it all the time. Skip the bath idea if you have kids like mine. We started to do bath time before dinner because of this.

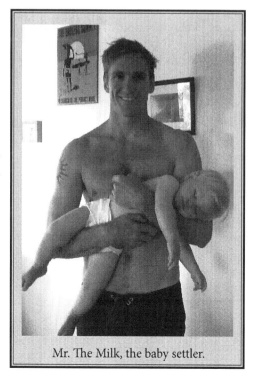

Mr. The Milk, the baby settler.

- **Books.** Reading to your child before bed (even as a new-born) is an excellent way to settle down and get relaxed. Cozy up together in your bed or on the couch and read some stories.
- **Massage.** Baby massage can work really well as a part of your routine, I mean who wouldn't want to be massaged prior to bed-time?! Sign me up!
- **Sing or put on some relaxing music.** Sing the same song every night to your child or put on some calm music.
- **Baby wearing.** Baby wearing can work really well during the night-time rituals as well as the nap times. It doesn't have to be you doing it! A family member, friend, or partner can help too if you have this support.
- **And of course… breastfeed!**

The basic underlying concept of all of this is that you can do these rituals around naps and bedtime and just boob the baby here or there, whenever they ask for it! This can be before, during, between or after the rituals. Continue to experiment with the things that work best for you and your baby and go with whatever works. If your baby starts to take longer to fall asleep or if the things that have been working suddenly fail, then it's time to change it up. Don't be surprised if breastfeeding eventually stops being that magical answer or if your baby just does not want to fall asleep in the baby carrier anymore. These changes are to be expected and it just requires a bit of creativity to find the next magical answer or group of activities that will do the trick. Most babies and toddlers will go through stages where boob just is not working! It could also be that your child is dropping one of his naps. Or maybe your toddler is dropping her day nap all together. This transition can be difficult but there does come a time where the nap patterns change, dropping from two to one and then completely. The age will vary but most babies and toddlers will continue to nap into their second or third year.

A BABY CRYING IS A BABY COMMUNICATING. PICK UP YOUR BABY, CUDDLE YOUR BABY, BREASTFEED YOUR BABY.

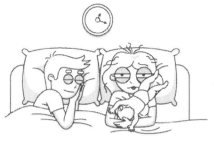

Co-Sleeping and Bedsharing Information

OK, let's first define co-sleeping and bedsharing. Many of us will use the term co-sleeping to describe when we sleep on the same mattress as our child. The definition of co-sleeping is to sleep in close proximity (and in the same room) with your baby, not actually WITH your baby. Bedsharing is sleeping with your child on the same sleeping surface.

No matter where or how your child sleeps there is always a risk of SIDS and suffocation, whether sleeping in a cot, bassinet, or bed. However, there are guidelines you can follow to decrease the risk. Co-sleeping and bedsharing are not dangerous in and of themselves. SIDS was formerly called "cot death" as babies who sleep in cots are also at risk of SIDS. While we cannot 100% remove the risks, we can follow safety guidelines to minimize them. The reality is that many of us who breastfeed on demand will at some point bring our babies and/or toddlers into bed with us. We find that we not only get more sleep, but our babies also tend to be happier and more settled as well. We all love a cuddle regardless of age so it's not a surprise that babies love it just as much as we do!

Since our babies are born so prematurely compared to other mammals, it is important for them to be close to us and have their needs immediately attended to (usually through breastfeeding and cuddling). Research shows that maternal smoking and inebriation are very significant risk factors when sleeping with your baby and therefore MUST be avoided. Breastfeeding is a protective factor against SIDS[1] and suffocation and every SIDS information booklet and website now includes breastfeeding as an important component in lowering your baby's risk.

It's really interesting to see how mothers and babies sleep together. Mothers will automatically sleep in a "cuddle curl" position. "Breastfeeding mothers instinctively protect their infants in their sleep. They adopt a cuddle curl position, and they touch and kiss their babies and adjust the baby's environment, often without waking. Breastfed babies instinctively stay in that protected cove."[2]

• Regardless of where your baby is sleeping (with you, near you or in their own room) it is VERY IMPORTANT that people in the house do not smoke as avoiding smoking has the biggest impact on preventing SIDS.[3]

• Breastfeed your baby

• Baby is full-term and healthy

• Do not sleep with your baby on a sofa or recliner as this is NOT a safe space to be sleeping with your baby.

• Alcohol free mother and non-drowsy medication only

• For those of you who are putting your baby to sleep in a cot, it is important that you have the cot free of toys, pillows, heavy blankets, and without bumpers along the sides.

• Don't put your baby to sleep on her stomach and without any heavy blankets.

• It is also important that your baby is not over-dressed for bed.

1. Australia's children 2002. Australian Institute of Health and Welfare. http://www.aihw.gov.au/WorkArea/DownloadAsset.aspx?id=6442459372. Published 2002. Accessed February 2, 2015.

2. Wiessinger, D., West, D., Smith, L.J., Pitman, T. *Sweet Sleep: Nighttime and Naptime Strategies for the Breastfeeding Family.* New York: Ballantine Books; 2014.

3. Bedsharing and safety. ISIS Infant Sleep And Information Source. https://www.dur.ac.uk/resources/isis.online/pdfs/ISIS_bedsharing_2014.pdf. Published 2014. Accessed April 9, 2015.

When looking at research on co-sleeping and bedsharing (or the statistics about SIDS), it's very important to differentiate between actual SIDS cases (where they are unexplained) and cases in which a baby has suffocated. A baby dying of suffocation is not supposed to be classified as SIDS. This can create results or statistics in a study that are not accurately reflective of the situation.

For further reading on research and evidence based information surrounding co-sleeping and bedsharing visit the Infant Information Source website which includes research from Dr. Helen Ball and Dr. James Mckenna's studies which can be found on his website, Mother-Baby Behavioral Sleep Laboratory. I also highly recommend the book, *Sweet Sleep* by Diane Wiessinger, Diana West, Linda J. Smith, and Teresa Pitman for La Leche League International. This book has a wealth of information to help you make informed decisions on how to go about sleeping with, or near your baby as safely as possible.

FAQs

When is the risk of SIDS greatest?

The risk of SIDS is greatest under 6 months of age, with a peak between 1–4 months old. Ninety percent of cases involve infants younger than 6 months.

Won't my partner squish my baby?

Mothers are connected to their baby's wake and sleep cycles since they are the ones waking and feeding their babies and are highly unlikely to squish their babies! As mentioned previously, it is also due to the "cuddle curl" position that mothers get into with their baby that protects the baby from being squished. Partners who are not breastfeeding are not as likely to be in this position. It is therefore safest to sleep between your baby and your partner. You can keep your baby from falling off the bed with a mesh toddler bed side rail. These can be found at most large retail outlets and baby stores. There are different styles available. When bedsharing, it is important to stuff the gap between the rail and the mattress with rolled up towels so it isn't a suffocation risk. You can also have a side car or co-sleeping bassinet that fits onto the side of your bed. For more information on co-sleeping and bedsharing options, continue on to the next chapter.

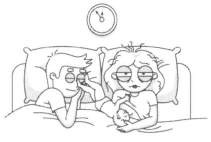

Co-Sleeping and Bedsharing Options for Your Family

Bedsharing and co-sleeping will not be for everyone, however the reality is that many of us around the world will sleep with (or very close) to our babies at some point or another, especially if we are breast-feeding. As we all know–some of us much more than oth-ers—breastfed babies tend to wake frequent-ly. Often, the closer we are to our babies, the more sleep we get!

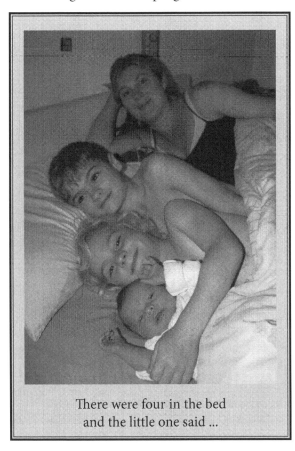

There were four in the bed
and the little one said ...

When we are pregnant, many of us don't give much thought to how we will (or will not) sleep with our babies. We are so focused on the birth that we usually just buy a cute little bassinet or cot and go from there. We might buy a little swaddling blanket or baby sleep sack but that's about it. We usually find that what we imagine ourselves doing when our babies arrive changes drastically once they are in our arms and on our breast.

My dear friend Emma was reflecting on the conversations she would have with people about this when pregnant with her first child: "People would ask me and I'd say, No! I'm definitely not going to sleep with my baby in the same bed. I'll squish him!"

However, when her baby arrived she quickly realized her feelings had changed: "Bringing him into our bed just felt like the right thing to do. It didn't feel right leaving him all alone in his room and I just knew I wouldn't squish him. Breastfeeding and co-sleeping; they were not things I consciously thought about, I just did it automatically."

There are many ways to co-sleep and bedshare and one size does not fit all. Even if you can follow the safe co-sleeping and bedsharing guidelines, you might find that it just does not work for you or that your little one really loves to sleep on her own (although I've never met one I'm assured they do exist!). Follow the lead of your baby. Do what works best for your child and for your family. It will be different for everyone. My youngest has always liked having his own space. We found that although he did not like to cuddle, he did like to be near us. My first two boys, however, were pretty much attached to me 24/7!

Ways to co-sleep (sleeping in the same room):

1. **Bassinet**

   There are endless options for bassinet styles! They can be put right next to your bed so you can easily sit up, reach over, and grab your baby.

2. **Side car or co-sleeper**

   This is the next step up toward more sleep! A co-sleeper attaches to the side of your bed. It has three sides so there is nothing between you and their little bed; it's like an extension of your own bed. This is great because you don't even have to sit up or move much to reach your baby. You can also cuddle up to them while still being on separate mattresses. Make sure you buy a rail that does not have a gap between the rail and the mattress, or put rolled up towels in the gap.

3. **Cot next to bed**

   If you have a cot you can bring this into your room (if you have the space) so that even though you are physically getting up out of bed, you are still in the same room as your baby.

4. **Cot turned co-sleeper**

   I know people who have turned their cots into co-sleepers! Many cots now have an option to move one of the sides all the way down. This can be very similar to the side car or co-sleeper option.

5. **Toddler bed**

   Once your baby is ready to move into a toddler bed, remember that you can continue to have your baby in your room with their little bed next to yours, before you move them into their own room. This can help with night-weaning as well. Most people agree that when your baby is around 18 months of age, you can start thinking about trying out the toddler bed (if you are ready for them to move into their own space). Of course, just make sure there is a side rail so they don't fall out!

Ways to bedshare (sleeping in the same bed):

1. **Baby between mother and side rail**

   Side rails are not just for toddler beds! An adjustable side rail can be used on an adult bed and then changed to a shorter rail when moved to a toddler bed. This will keep your baby from falling out of the family bed. Make sure you buy a rail that does not have a gap between the rail and the mattress or put a rolled towel in the gap.

2. **Baby in-between parents**

   A miniature baby bed can be positioned between the parents' pillows. These are a good alternative if you are not into cuddling all together in bed but still want your baby there.

3. **King size bed or room of mattresses**

   I know many families who do this! Forget the cute little bedroom interior design plan for the time being and just bring in the beds! Having a couple of mattresses on the floor can have you all together comfortably.

One of the most crucial parts of gentle, night-time mothering through breastfeeding is being flexible. What works one night might not work the next. This is completely normal and to be expected. Your baby might need extra cuddles or breastfeeds one night and then be completely happy to sleep in a bassinet for 6 hours straight the night after. If you are open to trying different options then night-time breastfeeding might be easier for you.

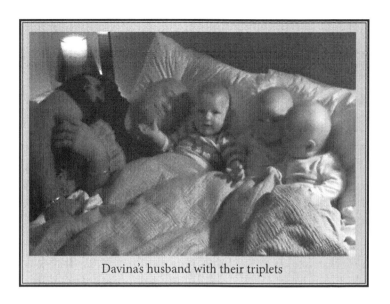
Davina's husband with their triplets

Davina, a mother of triplets (yes!) found a creative way to co-sleep and bedshare:

"When we first came home from the hospital the babies were 3 weeks old and we quickly realized that to maximise our sleep, the best plan for us was if daddy co-slept with two babies (the two slightly better sleepers) and I co-slept with one baby. When I woke to nurse my one, I would also pump and this would be the milk for daddy to feed the other two the next night. This plan worked so well for us, it continued until two of them slept through the night at 18 months old. The third was still waking for night-time boobie until he night-weaned himself at 2 years old. They are now 3 years old and only have night-time boobie if they are sick, or something has woken them up and they are upset. It felt like forever when we were in the middle of it, the constant night-waking, but letting them find their own path to sleeping through the night and night-weaning has meant that they are now all great sleepers, doing 12 hours straight through."

Remember that these sleeping arrangements will not last forever! Enjoy these cuddles with your babies and toddlers. Before you know it these moments will be gone. There will be a final breastfeed at 2am, the last cuddle as the sun rises, and the end of mothering through breastfeeding. These times can be challenging, but they are special. Changing how you sleep as a family can help with the challenging aspects.

And then sometimes this happens...

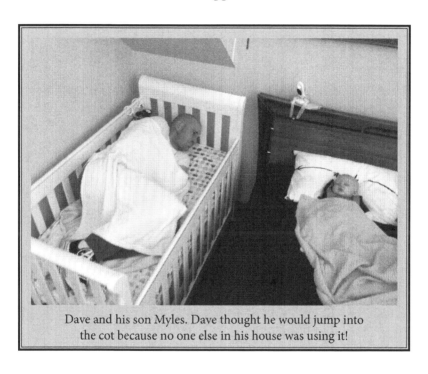

Dave and his son Myles. Dave thought he would jump into the cot because no one else in his house was using it!

SAFE BEDSHARING GUIDELINES

Smoking, intoxication, and not breastfeeding significantly increase the risk of SIDS and suffocation

When considering bedsharing it is important to have:

Healthy baby on his back, lightly dressed

Non-smoking, sober, breast-feeding mother

Both sleeping on a safe bed surface

* Co-sleeping and bedsharing will not work for everyone. Follow these guidelines, trust your instincts and follow the lead of your baby.

THE SAFE SLEEP SEVEN*

1. Smoke-free mother in and outside of the home

2. Alcohol and drug free mother, free from drowsy medications

3. Breastfeeding mother

4. Healthy, full-term baby

5. Baby not sleeping on his stomach.

6. Baby sleeps without heavy blankets and is lightly dressed

7. Safe bed surface, no bedsharing on couches or recliners

Babies older than four months can safely sleep with any sober, non-smoking adult on a safe bed surface.

*Adapted from *Sweet Sleep: Nighttime and Naptime Strategies for the Breastfeeding Family* by Diane Wiessinger, Diana West, Linda J. Smith, and Teresa Pitman for La Leche League International, Ballantine Books, 2014

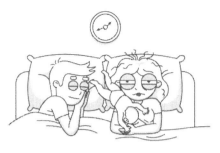

What to Do When Your Baby Hates to Sleep

Besides Drink Copious Amounts of Coffee

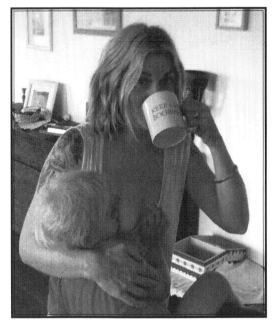

My youngest boy hates to sleep. And no, this is not just a little phase he is going through, nor is it my fault (although we do like to blame ourselves for these things). He has hated sleep from the second he was born all the way up until now (at just over 2 ½ years old).

You see, I have parented my three boys exactly the same. I breastfed them all to sleep, co-slept, and bedshared with them. I also held them often in a baby carrier, breastfed them well into toddlerhood (and beyond), and have pretty much mothered them through breastfeeding and cuddling the entire time. Yet they have all had very different sleep patterns. My middle boy literally loves to get into bed and fall asleep… always has and I imagine always will. I'm telling you all of this because #1. It's important to stop blaming yourself for your child's sleep issues. #2. You have not created your child's patterns. He is an individual who has different needs from the next baby. #3. Your baby's sleep issue is most likely not an issue at all, but simply normal… so stop believing

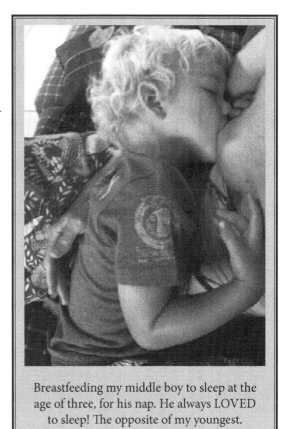

Breastfeeding my middle boy to sleep at the age of three, for his nap. He always LOVED to sleep! The opposite of my youngest.

all of those baby sleep books you are reading! "BUT! BUT!" you are yelling… I know. It's exhausting. It's annoying. It's downright torture dealing with little or no sleep.

So what did I do (and do I continue to do) about my youngest child who literally HATES to sleep? (*Just a side note here, I am all about responding to your child's needs through breastfeeds and/or cuddles. I also believe in following your own motherly instincts and your child's lead. This is the basic philosophy that I come from.) So this is it in a nutshell… my youngest still hates to sleep. The irony of all of this though is that he is taking a nap right now as I write this! HOWEVER, would you like to see the steps of how this nap actually happened?

• Carry a crying toddler down to the car. It's was an incredibly hot day so I wanted to see if a nice cool car ride in some air-conditioning would help. Believe me, I also wanted an excuse to sit in the AC as well! My oldest boy also had a friend over so there was no way the youngest was going to sleep with 3 boys in the house playing Legos.

- I wrestle a kicking, screaming toddler REFUSING to get into his car seat while I bake and sweat in the sun trying to force him in there like a ninja warrior.
- Ninja warrior defeated, I carry this crying toddler back up-stairs to my room.
- I hold him while he tantrums and cries and just patiently wait for him to stop tantruming in my arms and be ready to breastfeed again.
- He latches on and… silence. Eyes finally close and sleep finally happens.

Is it always this dramatic you might be asking? Well, no, sometimes he happily falls asleep breastfeeding. Other times he will fall asleep in the car on the way home from somewhere or he will just skip napping all together now that he is older. So let's get to some specifics on ways I have actually gotten my youngest to sleep! Because honestly… even when he was a baby it was not easy!

I recommend try-ing all or some of the following to get your baby to sleep and keep them asleep for a longer period of time… without hav-ing them cry it out.

- Breastfeed your child to sleep. Breast-feeding your child to sleep is not a bad hab-

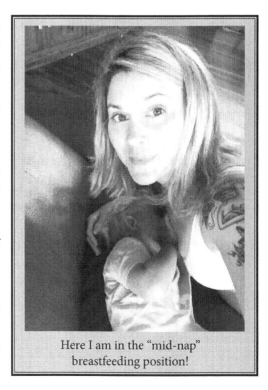

Here I am in the "mid-nap" breastfeeding position!

it. It is the biological norm and an awesome, calm, and loving way to put a child to sleep. Breastmilk contains components that help to put your baby to sleep.[1]

• Breastfeed your child the second they cry during a short nap (after the 30-40 minute cycle) to get them to fall back to sleep again for a longer nap. I call this the "mid-nap" breastfeeding position.

• Carry your child to sleep in the baby carrier. Remember you are now a marsupial!

• If possible, give your child to a friend, family member, or partner to carry or cuddle to sleep if boobin' does not work. When in doubt, whip it out! But sometimes the boob does not work. This is when getting some help is crucial for your sanity and your baby's sanity. Don't be afraid to ask for help. Historically, humans lived in tribal communities where they could pass their babies off to someone when they needed a break. This is because our babies are born so prematurely. They need constant cuddles and comfort.

• Sleep with him or near him following safe guidelines, so your baby can breastfeed during

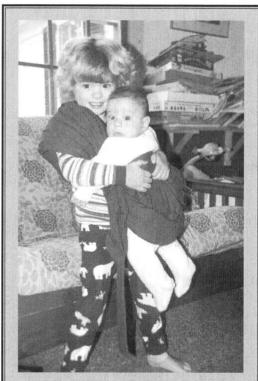

My oldest boy at the age of three practicing his baby wearing skills and finding his inner marsupial!

1. Sánchez C, Cubero J, Sánchez J, et al. The possible role of human milk nucleotides as sleep inducers. *Nutritional Neuroscience*. 2009; 12:2-8.

his nap and/or through the night. Many mothers find that by sleeping with or near their babies they can get more sleep.

• Even if your baby is waking frequently, you will not have to fully wake up to feed him as much as if he was in a different room.

• Let go of expectations of what normal is and stop comparing your baby to other children and how they sleep. Just like adults, they are all different. Find groups of women who mother like you do. This can really help, especially if you are starting to feel as though you are the only person in the world who mothers through breastfeeding and cuddling. There are millions of us out there! You just have to find us.

• Sit quietly with your baby skin-to-skin without people around. As your toddler gets older you can still do this (although she will be a bit more active!)

• Set some routines around nap-time and bed-time. You can still breastfeed on demand during your routines! It's not about scheduling breastfeeding/play/sleep times, but about putting some rituals into place that can be done before, during, or after breastfeeds leading up to nap-time or bed-time. Rituals can include reading books, going for a walk, or lying down quietly in your bed with them listening to some familiar music. I always sing the same two songs to my youngest when I'm breastfeeding him, trying to get him to sleep. Sometimes it actually works!

• Go with the flow and be adaptable to changing routines! Your baby or toddler will have times of being an awesome sleeper! Then they will start waking more frequently again. This is totally normal. My little guy takes naps still (although he does skip days) and will usually sleep for two hours. He did not do this regularly though until recently. I have no idea why he suddenly started taking longer naps… we just go with it!

One of the most important aspects of a baby's changing sleep patterns is to recognize our expectations (or the expectations of those around us) and what is seen as a sleep problem or something that must be changed or fixed. Breastfed babies and toddlers are not meant to sleep through the night, and there are

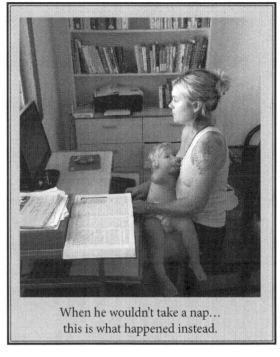

When he wouldn't take a nap…
this is what happened instead.

many reasons for this. If we can just change our outlook about this and get back to basics! Think of yourself as a marsupial, not a mammal. Carry your baby, breastfeed your baby frequently, and just plain cuddle him and comfort him! This is what most babies and toddlers need. Babies and toddlers do not need to be fixed or trained. It's us and our lifestyles that need some fixin'.

My baby hated sleep and did not settle easily, however he was not distressed. If you have a baby who cries a lot or is clearly not sleeping because he is uncomfortable, in pain or colicky, please contact me or another lactation consultant who can help you get to the bottom of it. Sometimes sleep issues can be caused by specific medical or gut-related issues, such as food intolerances or allergies.

BREASTFEEDING
TO SLEEP...
BREASTFEEDING
TO AWAKE...
BREASTFEEDING
TO CALM...
BREASTFEEDING
TO COMFORT.

NOT A PROP.
NOT A HABIT.

THE BIOLOGICAL NORM

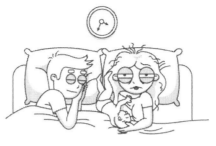

The Transition Boob

How to keep your baby asleep while moving them to a different area...

We have all been through this before. Our child falls asleep peacefully while in the car or out for a walk and then we cringe while we try to figure out how to move her. Or maybe your baby falls asleep peacefully at the breast but then wakes up the second your try to put her down! My son WOULD NOT let me put him down. Anywhere. The second I went to put him on his back, his little eyes would pop open! Folks, this is when you can try what I have coined, the "transition boob." This is appropriate for a baby if you have a co-sleeper or cot which is directly in contact with your bed, for an older child who can sleep with a toddler rail on the

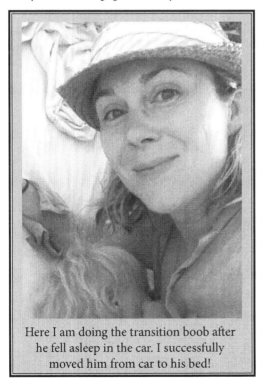

Here I am doing the transition boob after he fell asleep in the car. I successfully moved him from car to his bed!

side of a mattress, or if you are going to bedshare following safe guidelines.

So here is the basic idea of how the transition boob works. You pick your baby up from wherever they have fallen asleep (pram, car, partner's lap) and you pop him straight onto the breast. This will usually settle him back into a deep (or deep-ISH) sleep. Keep breastfeeding while carefully moving to your desired final sleep spot for your child. The easiest way to make this transition is on a sleeping surface you can both lie down on together. Once you are on the mattress with them get into the side lying nursing position and breastfeed until they are settled and you can try de-latching. Now this is where you may have to use the "comfort hold" as I like to call it. This picture demonstrates what I am talking about…

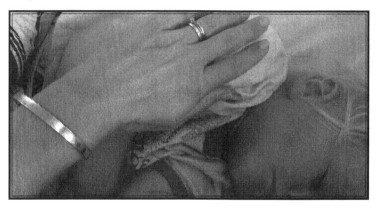

Pretty much it just involves you gently but firmly resting your hand on their arm. This has worked brilliantly for all of our children during the transition! It is usually only necessary to do as you de-latch them from your breast and then move carefully away from them. You may need to attempt this a few times before your child eventually stays settled. It can help your child feel that sense of security as they go from breastfeeding to sleeping without you there. It is of course important to do this while following safe sleep guidelines. I know of quite a few people who have done this while lying in their child's cot! It is actually possible, although it would be much easier to do this with a co-sleeper attached to your bed. Rest with your baby as much as you can. Instead of getting up to do the dishes have a quick rest.

As your child gets older, it will become easier and easier to accomplish the transition. My youngest (who at the time of finishing up this book is still breastfeeding at 2 ½) will now very happily de-latch when I put him in his bed at night. You will not need to do the transition boob forever! Of course when your baby is little you can try to transition her to a new sleeping spot without breastfeeding to see how she responds to it. The transition boob method might work well for you though if you find that your baby does not respond well to a transition without breastfeeding.

Now I know exactly what some people might be thinking right now, particularly if they are a sleep-trainer or cry-it-out/self-settling/pick-up-put-down baby sleep person. "This all sounds ridiculous! It seems like it would be so much easier to just go through a few days of your baby crying then to do this for the entire time they're breastfeeding." I totally get why people might say this, but here's the thing… none of my boys responded well to just being put down and falling asleep on their own. They all wanted my cuddles, wanted to breastfeed, and just needed that physical contact to fall (and stay) asleep. It did not feel right letting them cry. I was following my instincts and the lead of my babies and I'm OK with that. I'm OK with meeting my children's needs this way and mothering through cuddles and breastfeeds. If you feel the same as I do, then this might be helpful for you too! Trust your instincts and follow the lead of your baby, not what someone else thinks is best, but what you feel is best for you and your family.

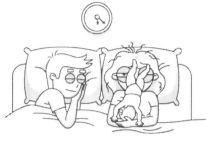

What About My Partner?

Combining Gentle Parenting with a Partnership

We have all heard the naysayers and negative nellies in regards to attachment parenting and how to combine it successfully with a marriage or partnership. "But when do you actually have sex?!… You can't possibly find time for each other with your toddler attached to your boob 24/7! We need to go out together at least once a week without the kids." So what keeps relationships alive? How is it possible to breastfeed on demand, co-sleep or bedshare, wear your baby almost constantly, delay going anywhere together without children for at least the first six to nine months, breastfeed them to sleep, take care of them while awake and everything in-between, while still having the energy, time, and desire to actually want to hang out with another human being? The good news is… it's possible. It's not only possible but with a little creativity, communication, and attention to detail, your marriage can not only survive but flourish… and you might even be able to find extra time to have sex. Or go out to coffee together, that's almost the same thing right?!

What can we do to help our partners understand? One of the most important things we can do is help them to see why it's so important that we be close to our nurslings at night. This is what my husband has to say on this:

> "As animals, the human design sucks. Every other mammal has only a few moments to get on its feet and then it hangs with the pack. Mum looks

after the young ones and dad looks after the herd. Humans are useless in a kinaesthetic sense; the main focus is on developing an awesome brain. One thing in common though is that mother's milk is key. It is vital and it is the foundation from which these animals (humans included) grow, survive, and eventually reproduce themselves. At the end of the day our main job is to reproduce and make sure our offspring make it to that age to do the same. We may have grand plans for young Johnny or Jessie in the future, but those first few months and years are the most crucial... what better way to start than by being snuggled up with mum and dad while having milk on tap."

Remember those romantic, love story movies that make married life look like all fun and games? Well let's start by being honest here... relationships are HARD WORK (A special thanks to my mother for telling me this right before I got married. Every single person needs this little fairy tale bubble to be burst before they get into a long term relationship). My husband and I have been together for fifteen years. We have three children ranging from almost 3 to 11 years old. We had our first baby while we were finishing college. For about six months we lived with my parents after our baby was born. We were broke, newlyweds, and I was breastfeeding while finishing my degree. We co-slept with our baby, I was never away from him and I was exhausted (as all of us new mums are, regardless if

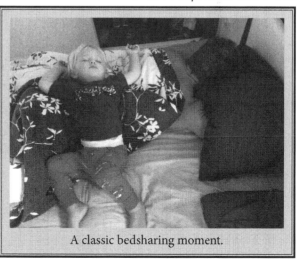

A classic bedsharing moment.

we are breastfeeding or not). So how did we survive this incredibly challenging start and manage to still be married a decade later? We work EVERY. SINGLE. DAY. to keep our relationship going.

Disclaimer I am not a marriage counselor. I am not a spiritual advisor. I am a mum of three who has been married for awhile. We have fought, we have made up, we have cried together, we have laughed together, and somehow are still standing together. Take from this what you feel might work for you and your relationship… leave the rest behind.

I'd like to start with the list my husband came up with for this article.

1. Have sex

2. Repeat step one

The End.

He did go on to say this though!

> "Often dads and even myself, do, or have, worried about certain things. Like during pregnancy we worry that we'll hurt the baby during sex. Well now that the little bugger has survived that, what about sex in the place where it possibly all began? People, where there is a will, there is a way. And any dads out there whose will is as strong as mine, you'll know that it means be proactive. Maybe set the cot next to the bed or a little mattress that will make it an easy transition for when the horizontal monkey dance is finished and the little one gets fussy. Also think about different rooms, different times of day (rather than at night when mum is tired and baby is cranky)."

Gentle/Attachment parenting and our partners... how to combine the two?

1. How will we ever get to go out and get away from the kids? Let go of the idea that there is a step-by-step guide to life that we must follow. Date for an appropriate amount of time, get married, go on a honeymoon, have a baby, etc. etc. Most people get married and then go on a honeymoon. When we got married we had a three-month-old, so did we just throw out the whole thing altogether? No! We went on our honeymoon when our baby weaned at 2 years and three months old. It was awesome and we really appreciated that time together. The next childless trip we went on was a long weekend in Perth. This was before I was pregnant with #3 and baby #2 was about four years old. Weaned and totally fine without us for a few days... with no parent guilt at all!

2. But we really want to go out to dinner! Think morning time. Forget going out to dinner just the two of you for the first year (at least) unless you want to pump and have someone else put them to bed. When I have a nursling who is under the age of two and not yet night-weaned, my husband and I go out to breakfast or an early dinner. I'm talking 5 pm, people! Yes, we are out with the families with kids and elderly people but at least we are childless! You can laugh and empathize with the other poor souls who are there mopping up spilled drinks and running after their children. It is totally possible to have fun with the kids too. Try to go out together at least once per week. Even if you have to bring your little minion with you as we did here while getting a coffee. Our oldest two were in school and my husband had the day off so we went to the local coffee shop!

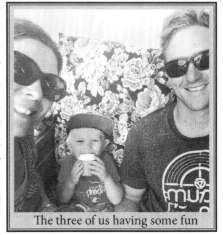
The three of us having some fun

3. Fight. And then make up. Yes this step sounds a little weird, but if you fight FAIR then it can be a great way of communicating. Remember to make up though. Bake him a cake, have him bake you a cake, have sex, or give him a hug. Whichever you prefer at the time…

Fighting fair means doing the following…

Identify clearly how you feel, if you need time to yourself then say it and walk away, let your partner walk away if they need to, stay on the subject, do not bring up past fights or circumstances, don't say mean or untrue things. If fighting in front of your kids refrain from yelling and make up in their presence as well (even if it's some time later) so they can see how the process works. Remember it is hard to hug a porcupine, so try not to be a porcupine. Or an echidna if you live in Australia.

4. Having a baby on your boob 24/7 is extremely exhausting… how will I have time to do anything else?! When you are feeling touched out, TELL YOUR PARTNER YOU ARE FEELING TOUCHED OUT! Sometimes as breastfeeding mothers we just feel so frustrated and really not in a need of a cuddle but we cannot put our finger on exactly what is going on… this could be it. There were times I felt totally touched out. After having a child attached to my boob 24/7 there were nights where I just could not even bear to think of touching anyone else! Not even a hug! When I feel this way, I tell my husband. Then he knows where I'm coming from. Yes it sounds simple but we often want our partners to read our minds when in fact they cannot. Unless they are psychic… in which case they should be on TV making millions of dollars and helping to solve crimes in their spare time.

5. Talk about how your relationship has changed and how you feel about it. The days are gone when you were having sex 24/7 and had time to go out to dinner, talk about your day without being interrupted 46 times, and could go for a walk on the beach without a crying kid on one side of you and an older child complaining that they are bored. You are still in an awesome relationship, just a different awesome relationship.

6. Sex does not have to occur after dinner and the evening news, in your bed and after a thorough teeth brushing between 8:30 and 10pm. Brad Pitt once spoke about how he and Angelina Jolie would put on a movie during the day for the kids and sneak off into the bedroom. It's all about creativity! If you really have the need to be in your bed then temporarily move your baby or toddler into a bassinet, cot, or mattress on the floor. To imply that attachment parents never have sex or must have difficulty because of co-sleeping or bedsharing with their kids, we'd need to wonder about those who keep having children past the first-born… it's not from immaculate conception.

7. Show interest in what your partner has to say, even when your baby is crying, your toddler is pooping in the closet, and all you can think about is sleep. My husband and I will readily admit to each other sometimes we are so bored out of our minds listening to the other person go on and on and we are often distracted by the kids. For my husband, the boring subject he must listen to is of course… breastfeeding! But he knows that if he can at least pretend to be interested then I'm happy! This might sound ridiculous and horrid to a newlywed couple, but believe me. If your partner is taking the time to pretend to be interested there is effort being put in and that means something. Most of the time of course we are interested… but sometimes we are not! When my husband starts to go on about cricket or rugby, my eyes glaze over… but I try. I really, really try. Most of the time.

8. Get some me time in. As frequently as possible. You might be thinking, but what does this have to do with my relationship? It has EVERYTHING to do with your relationship! You cannot function in an adult relationship without taking care of yourself and getting your own time. Sometimes for me this means just ten minutes by myself (possibly with my almost two-year-old asking for me on the other side of the door with my husband trying to distract him with crackers or trains). Ten minutes by yourself can literally change your entire day! Your partner needs me time too. Let's be real here folks, men tend to be able to take time to themselves with little or no guilt while us mums feel insane amounts of guilt for taking some time for ourselves… let me just say, get over it and go do something without someone latched onto your boob!

9. Talk about what needs to change SPECIFICALLY to help things go smoother with day-to-day stuff. My husband used to work out after he got home from work. You know that time of day when your older kids are going crazy running around fighting and your baby is wanting to breastfeed CONSTANTLY while you are trying to cook dinner? This was the worst time for me. We talked about this and he changed when he works out. Now he goes before work or does some exercise in the garage while our toddler hangs out with him. I get to cook dinner by myself while he works out! Win win for all… kind of. Exercising with a toddler is not all it's cracked up to be.

10. Patience. When you are out of baby world you will all of a sudden realize certain milestones… "I just read three pages of a book without being interrupted or falling asleep!" "I just ate an entire meal in silence!" Or, "I slept in past 7 am! Without having to take my boob out!" These times will come.

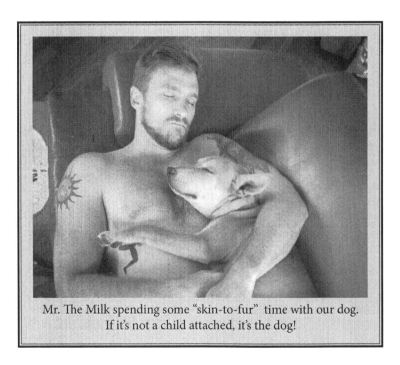

Mr. The Milk spending some "skin-to-fur" time with our dog.
If it's not a child attached, it's the dog!

11. Meeting the needs of your children through attachment parenting and breastfeeding does not mean ignoring your own needs or the needs of your partner. Attachment parenting at the expense of your other relationships helps no one, especially your kids. Teach your kids the importance of taking the time to nurture ALL of your relationships, beyond the parent-child one.

12. Your baby will need you 24/7. Yes, we can have it all. We can have a great marriage, a baby, and a career. But we cannot do this all at once. We cannot have it all, all at once. Mothering through breastfeeding means being with your baby. When we are in it we feel exhausted, overwhelmed, and sometimes plain bored. We need adult conversation, we need to get out, we need a break. You can do all of this while still breastfeeding on demand and paying attention to your husband over there in the corner who is looking at you with those big sad eyes… "Remember me?" but those first few months it will be mostly focused on your baby. And that's OK.

13. It is dangerous thinking that you can pay attention to your relationship with your partner after the kids have grown up. Don't believe it for a second. It takes communication and effort along the way… but give yourself a break those first few months and love up that new little baby of yours.

It is possible to successfully combine gentle parenting with a partnership! It just takes some attention and creativity.

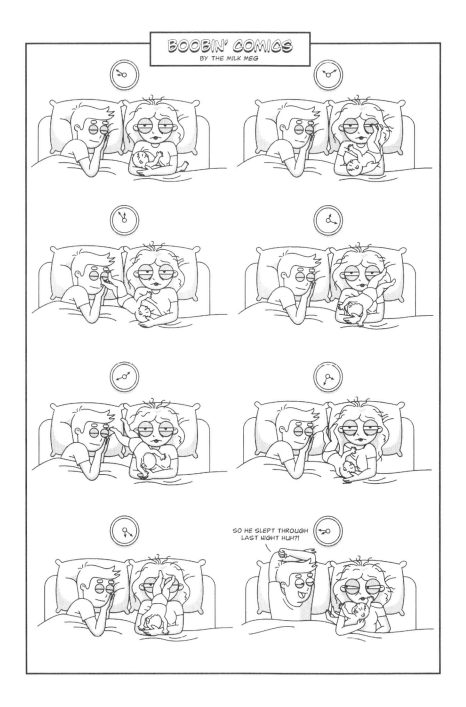

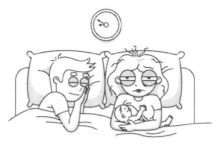

Coffee! Can I Still Drink Coffee?!

Since I'm writing about how exhausted we all are, I have to include a chapter about coffee, right?! Sitting and drinking a cup of coffee is my happy place. I gaze dreamily at my mug following a marathon pre-dawn early morning boobin' session and can't wait to drink it! Of course many of us worry about the caffeine that's in our wonderful little (or big) cup of coffee and if it's going to go through our milk and affect our baby. Thankfully most of us can drink a cup or two without any issues.

Medications and Mother's Milk, the awesome and ever-so-informative book by Thomas Hale, is my go-to book for information on medications and lactation. Believe it or not, caffeine is used as a medication and is sometimes given to premature babies as a treatment for breathing problems. The dose given is much higher than what is found in mother's milk after caffeine consumption.[1]

The reality is that caffeine is commonly consumed by both pregnant and lactating women. I mean seriously, how are we supposed to function without it?! Studies show that for most women, moderate consumption of caffeine will not affect their babies. One study concluded that caffeine consumption during pregnancy and by nursing mothers seems to not have any consequences on the sleep of infants at three months of age.[2]

---

1   Breastfeeding and caffeine. Kellymom. http://kellymom.com/bf/can-i-breastfeed/lifestyle/caffeine/ Published July 29, 2011. Accessed January 9, 2015.

2   Santos IS, Matijasevich A, Domingues MR. Maternal caffeine

It is important to note that the half-life of coffee decreases with the age of your baby. In neonates (newborns) it is as high as 97.5 hours but decreases to 14 hours at 3–5 months and 2.6 hours at 6 months and older.[3] This means that as babies get older, it takes less time for their bodies to process caffeine and get it out of their systems. Some women will wait a few months following the birth of their baby to start drinking caffeine again because of this. My friend Emily tried drinking a cup of coffee when her breastfed baby was about 3 months old. He was WIDE AWAKE for almost the entire day and she was hyper as well! This is because she had not had coffee in almost one year... so they both had a strong reaction to it! When she waited a few months and tried coffee again, she found that it did not have any affect on the baby's sleep at all and she could start to drink it regularly.

The key point to remember is that the older your baby is, the less likely caffeine will affect him or her. But please drink it in moderation! What does that mean? Your baby will let you know! Caffeine may affect some younger babies but for others it won't be a problem. Try to limit your intake to 1 or 2 cups per day and always observe your baby for signs on whether your caffeine consumption is working for them or not.

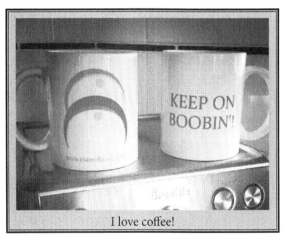
I love coffee!

consumption and infant nighttime waking: prospective cohort study. *Pediatrics*. 2012; 129(5):860-8. doi: 10.1542/peds.2011-1773.

3   Hale T. *Medication and Mother's Milk*. 14th ed. St Amarillo, Texas: Hale Publishing; 2010.

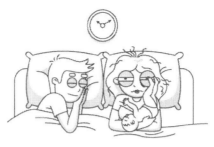

How Do I Get My Baby to Take Longer Naps?

Around the time my youngest was about 7 months old, he suddenly decided he did not want to nap for longer than thirty minutes. He would look like this picture, so peaceful and dreamy… and then he would wake up. He would wake up either a. happy as could be or b. upset and wanting to breastfeed, but after breastfeeding he would be wide awake and happy.

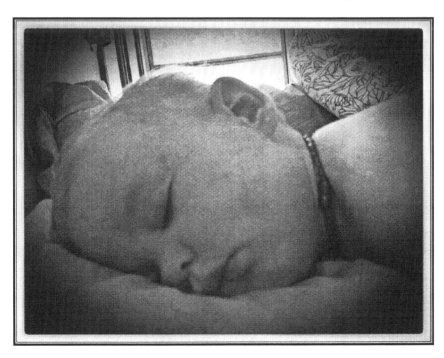

I either a. cried or b. vented to my husband each night about the complete and total exhaustion I was feeling because of it. He would then sleep in thirty- to ninety-minute chunks at night.

READ: I WAS NOT GETTING MORE THAN ONE AND A HALF HOURS OF UNINTERRUPTED SLEEP FOR TWO WEEKS STRAIGHT!

Here is an illustration I drew of how I was feeling during this time… as you can see I'm an awesome artist.

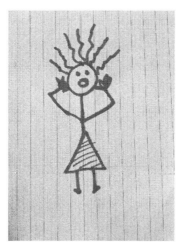

I was also getting ready to have 8 people over for Christmas Day. This is how I felt on Christmas Day from lack of sleep…

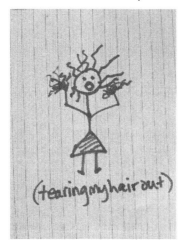

(tearing my hair out)

When the first lot of relatives arrived for Christmas lunch I was still in my PJs and had not showered yet!

Now I am thankfully back to normal, as my youngest has decided to start napping again! Yay for me! This is the natural, cyclical nature of babies and sleep.

We are all looking for that magical answer… how do I get my baby to nap longer during the day? Here is the magical answer… I actually have no idea what the magical answer is! This is because EVERY BABY IS AN INDIVIDUAL! Yes, I mention this throughout my book because so often we forget this and many baby books do not acknowledge this. There is no one answer that will work for everyone, all of the time, UNLESS crying is involved. However, I do have some tips that have worked for me at various times with various babies to get them to nap longer. Does it always work? No. But many times it does! Then I rejoice and have some peace and quiet during the day for a bit longer to do all of those exciting things we parents at home get to do… laundry, cooking, cleaning, going to the toilet, and occasionally getting to eat while sitting down.

Here are my top tips!

1. First and foremost, breastfeed your baby back to sleep if they wake up after a short nap. With my eldest boy I would lie down with him on my bed just as he would start to stir or cry. This way he would just barely wake up before I could quickly breastfeed him back to sleep. This works great if they really don't want to be awake yet. Sometimes he would then fall back asleep for another hour or two! You can put a single or toddler mattress on the floor (and add mesh toddler rails for safety) so that you can easily hop onto and off of the bed and avoid having your child roll off the high bed onto the floor!

2. Routine, routine, routine! Rituals, rituals, rituals! I remember asking my paediatrician about naps when I was a new mum. "What is normal?" I asked him. He simply said, "It's totally up to the parents whether or not babies and kids take naps." I didn't really get it at the time, but three kids later I can see what he means. If you create regular rituals in your child's day, he or she will fall into those routines easily and be more likely to nap and stay asleep. With the first child it's easier. By the time numbers 2 and 3 come along, it can get more difficult due to driving around for schedules and appointments like a crazy woman throughout the day! Some days your baby can take a nap in the car or while being carried around in a carrier. This is not only OK, but expected, especially after you have had a few kids.

3. Sometimes your baby's nap will happen during a long breastfeed. Even though many of us (myself included) would prefer to have some time during the day by ourselves without a little creature attached to us, sometimes this just doesn't happen. It's totally normal to have those days when babies will only sleep while breastfeeding or being held. Allowing the time to do this is important. Cuddles through baby wearing, hugging, and breastfeeding are wonderful (and I would argue crucial) for the well-being of our little ones.

4. Keep this mantra in your head, "Once I reach my breaking point, my baby will change and all will be peaceful again!" My mother told me this one and boy is it true. At times your baby/toddler/child will bring you to the point of insanity (see above illustrations) and you will think, "I can't do this anymore! I must sleep! My child must sleep!" They stop taking short naps and all of a sudden start marathon naps and night sleeps. This has happened to me many times over the years. I am happy to report that soon after writing this, my little cherub suddenly decided to take amazingly long daytime naps and sleep in 3–4 hour chunks at night! Hooray! Hooray! Hooray! This is how I feel now…

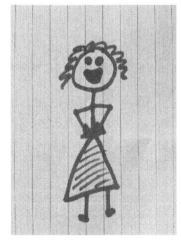

5. Remind yourself that babies have these variations in daytime (and night-time) sleep for many different reasons. After those two crazy weeks, I realized that my little guy was getting another tooth! The poor thing was in pain and probably as exhausted as me. I feel great, though, knowing that during this time I breastfed him, cuddled him, and slept by his side as he needed it. Other times I realized after a difficult stretch that he was getting sick. Also, sometimes babies change their sleep patterns when they are going through a developmental milestone such as learning to roll over or crawl. Regardless of the reason, it's just about being there for them.

6. Often my baby will not go down for a nap unless I carry him around in my baby carrier. He will fall asleep in the carrier and then we go through this little routine to get him to finally nap…

- take him out of the carrier and he wakes up
- breastfeed him back to sleep
- put him down and he wakes up again
- breastfeed him back to sleep
- put him down again and he sleeps! Yay! My hard work pays off eventually.

Then all was happy and peaceful… until something else changed and it all started again! The cycle of parenting…

*It is recommended that children are placed on their backs to sleep, to help prevent SIDS. At the time this photo was taken, my son was rolling onto his stomach on his own after he had fallen asleep.

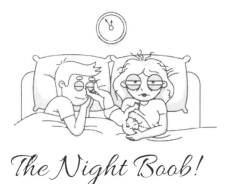

The Night Boob!

How To Gently Night-Wean Your Toddler From Breastfeeding And Bedsharing

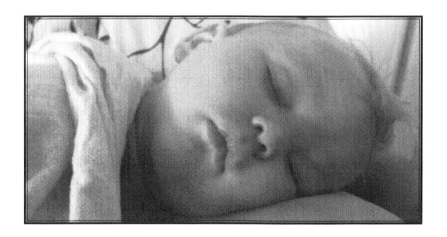

Many of us breastfeeding mothers go through the same stages of night time boobing...

1. We have our baby and listen to our instincts which for lots of us include: breastfeeding on demand, breastfeeding to sleep, breastfeeding to awake, breastfeeding during the night (possibly one thousand times) co-sleeping and/or bed sharing and generally having our baby on our boob or hip most of the time.

2.　We learn to ignore comments thrown at us frequently from strangers, family, and friends. Some examples: "She will NEVER learn to fall asleep on her own!" or "You are spoiling her!" or "You will never get her out of your bed!" We learn how to ignore those who boast, "Wow, my baby has been sleeping through for the past three months! Are you sure it's normal your baby is still waking?" The seeds of doubt are then planted in our minds, but we continue to breastfeed at night, holding onto our own instincts and what we feel is best.

3.　We continue happily with breastfeeding through the night, thankful for the easy and convenient way we can settle our babies, while still getting some rest ourselves. It's all so wonderful! Yes we are tired, but we are passionate about mothering through breastfeeding!

4.　Then we start to pass into the dark side of night boobing! We become exhausted, frustrated and generally at the point of wanting to cry, actually crying, or starting to doubt what we have done up to this point. We are torn between wanting to continue to meet the night-time needs of our babies, and wanting our boobs back! We want more sleep! Our baby is now a toddler who takes up more room, breastfeeds as frequently (or more frequently)than a newborn and yells, "Mama!" "Boobie!" or "Milk!" at us throughout the night. Our happy little co-sleeping families become a bit cranky and unsure of how to move ahead. How can I night-wean? How can I get her out of our bed without having her cry? I'm so confused!

Night-waking is the biological norm, but many of us get to the point where we just cannot go on like this! If you are happy continuing to breastfeed at night, awesome! Keep on going and read a different chapter. If you would like some ideas on how to night-wean and get your child sleeping in his own bed, then please keep reading.I will suggest some ideas that I have heard from other mothers, along with my suggestions and thoughts on the whole subject. I have successfully night-weaned three

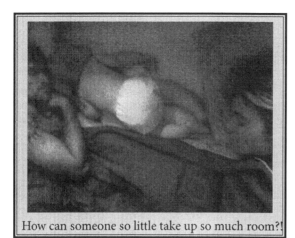
How can someone so little take up so much room?!

children. My first two boys were night-weaned just after they turned two and my third at the age of two-and-a-half years old. My experiences were different for all three boys. My suggestions are not as black-and-white as you will find in many other sleep books, but you will find different suggestions to try to see what works best for you and your child. THIS GUIDE IS NOT STEP BY STEP! Be wary of the 6 steps to getting your baby to sleep books. This means that for some (many) babies, they will cry as you move through those steps. My philosophy is to try different ideas and do what works best for you! There is no one-size fits-all approach to gentle night-weaning.

We want our boobs back at night, but we want the transition to be as peaceful as possible...

First things first!

If at ANY time you feel as though your toddler is really not ready for night-weaning, or instinctively you feel as though it's not the right thing to do, then STOP doing it and go back to what feels right for you and your child. You know your child best!

If your child is younger than 18 months old, I do not recommend attempting these strategies unless it feels like the right timing for you and your child, and she is responding well. If she cries for five seconds and then calms down and falls asleep, then maybe she is ready for this a bit earlier than others. Go with what your instincts and your child are telling you. At 18 months old, most toddlers can understand what you are saying and you can negotiate with them. It is all about meeting your child where she is at developmentally. Some will be ready earlier than others. From a developmental perspective, most children at about 18 months old are able to not only understand what you are saying to them, but can also communicate with you to some extent—with a few words, or with many. This is crucial to gentle night-weaning.

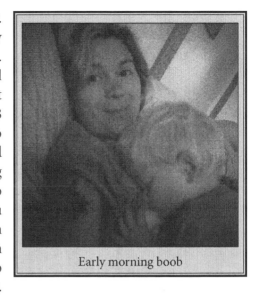

Early morning boob

Your child being able to communicate with you is so important for a gentle approach to night-weaning. You are working through this with a child who can understand what is happening and can express to you what he is feeling about it. He may not like it, but at least at this age they can understand what is happening. Try this at two months old and you will have a completely different experience. Babies cannot communicate except through crying and they cannot understand why we would deny them the boob!

My friend Emily was able to gently night-wean her little boy a couple of months after his first birthday. She could see that he was ready for it even though he was still quite young:

> "It was just after Oliver was about 13 months old when I noticed that he had started to wean himself off one to two of his day time breastfeeds. Although he had always been a big eater and had been breastfed on demand since day one, he started to show less interest in his mid-morning and mid-afternoon feeds. Up until this point he was still feeding up to two, sometimes three times during the night and was sleeping in his cot in his own room. I made the choice to attempt night-weaning mainly due to the fact that I was extremely run

down and had been diagnosed with ross river fever so I was far from 100%, and most importantly, I felt comfortable that Oliver was ready for this step. I first altered his bedtime routine slightly by not breastfeeding him to sleep, by feeding him in the lit lounge room not in his room, and followed this by a bedtime story (I used to do this the other way around in his dimmed room). I truly didn't think he would work with my plan as he was a big breastfeeder, but after about a week of gently changing this routine he was happy to go to sleep without my boob. Once I had changed this routine he seemed to wake less. If he did wake I gave him a sippy cup of warm expressed breast milk which I gradually watered down. I was dreading this process and yet Oliver pleasantly surprised me! I don't think I would have been comfortable night-weaning him any earlier as I'm not sure he would have been entirely ready for the process. Although he was night-weaned, he was always very ready for a breastfeed around 5am! He is now 17 months and still wakes during the night from time to time, mainly if he is teething or feeling unwell, and I simply give him his water bottle, which he loves, or a sippy cup of warm goat's or cow's milk."

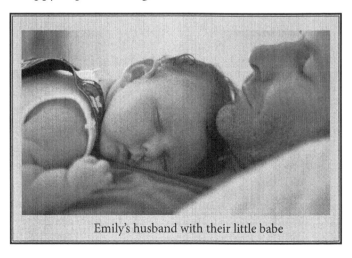

Emily's husband with their little babe

This approach is for a child who is healthy and parents who agree that this is best and are supporting each other. If your child has health issues going on, maybe night-weaning is not the best option for you. If your partner does not support this process then you might find it is more difficult... not impossible of course, but could be more difficult.

You can choose to try all of these steps, one of these, or a combination. It's all about what feels best for you. Nothing about the gentle process of night-weaning and encouraging them to sleep in their own beds is black and white.

You cannot see this as a linear process. It's two steps forward, one step back for many of us... and then possibly one step to the side and up! This will not happen overnight and might not happen for a few weeks or months depending on how slow you would like to take it.

Remember your child has been sleeping with you and your boobs for their whole little life! Although we want it to happen quickly, it often takes time as they are getting used to a completely different way of falling and staying asleep, which they have never had to do until this point. Patience on your part is incredibly important. Remember our gentle parenting mantra?

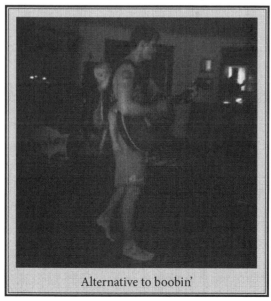

Alternative to boobin'

The Milk Meg's Collection of Night Boob Weaning Ideas!

THE MOST IMPORTANT PART OF THIS PROCESS...

Communicate with your child. Start talking to them about the difference between day and night. Take them outside and show them the moon and stars at night and the sunshine during the day. Talk about how we sleep at night and we wake when the sun shines. This is CRUCIAL to do before and during this process. Even at twelve months old your child can start to understand day and night and most can speak in a one-word sentence. By eighteen months your child has telegraphic speech where they have subject-object sentences.[1] This is the basis for this entire process. We are explaining to them that night-time is for sleep (when the moon is up and stars are out) and daytime is for being awake and of course, for boobies!

You can discuss the difference between day and night and "boobies when the sun shines, not when the moon is out" for days, weeks, or months before you start trying out the night-weaning suggestions. It is up to you and how you are feeling about your child's readiness and understanding. I would recommend talking about it a few times per day though before you start. Consistency is key!

Idea #1 Having your partner, friend or family member put your child to bed (instead of your boob).

Some toddlers are 100% about boobing to sleep. They will not fall asleep any other way and will get extremely upset without breastfeeding. If this sounds like your little one, idea #1 might not be the best approach to take. Yet, there are many little munchkins out there who will happily fall asleep while being cuddled or carried by someone other than mum. This is a good way to start transitioning them off the boob for falling asleep. Instead of breastfeeding your little one to sleep, hand her over to your partner or well-loved (by your child) family member or friend to put her to sleep instead. This could be through rocking,

---

1. Riordan J, Wambach K. *Breastfeeding and Human Lactation.* 3rd ed. Jones and Bartlett: Boston; 2010.

singing, lying down with them in their beds, or rubbing their backs. If you do not have someone else to help you, you can try this yourself. REGARDLESS OF WHO IS DOING THIS, COMMUNICATE WITH THE TODDLER! Explain to her very clearly before you put her to bed that this is what is going to happen. "Daddy is going to put you to bed. No booby tonight." You will find that by not breastfeeding to sleep, they are more likely (over time) to stop waking to breastfeed during the night. *Note: Over time… not straight away! Unless you have lucky fairy dust surrounding you and have won the night-time lottery.

Here is Karen's story about night-weaning her 20-month-old twins:

> "Through talking to Meg I learned how to talk with my twins about night-weaning and that due to them now being 20 months old, their level of understanding was great enough for it to be a gentle process. As it was winter we couldn't really look out of the window in the morning and look at the sunshine as a cue for milk. So I bought a special clock which shows children night and day, using a star and a sun. I chose for the sun to come up at 6 am. For three nights we read a children's book about night-weaning and I talked to them about the moon and stars how 'boobies go to sleep.' We talked about the clock as well as looking out of the window. They clearly understood as Ellis began to show he didn't like the clock and Reuben wasn't sure about the book.
>
> When the day came to change the routine, we started to talk about the day and night and how boobies go to sleep. They settled to sleep in the cots as normal. When they woke in the night I used whatever method I could (apart from feeding) to settle them back to sleep. We cuddled, sang, played music, and looked at books. They even started to pick out the children's book I had

about night-weaning! Ellis found the transition harder, and personality-wise I had expected that. For the first two nights he would spend time nearly every night walking around the room and crying. But it wasn't a sad cry. He was angry. This helped me stay with what we were doing. After about 2 1/2 weeks, Reuben slept until 4 am and after 3 weeks until 5 am. Ellis still woke more often but eventually he too made it until 4 am!

They are yet to 'sleep through' and I am yet to spend a night in the same bed as my husband. But we have made significant progress. And it has been gradual and gentle. There are still nights with wakes before 4 am, but they are both easily settled back to sleep with a cuddle on my mattress, and sometimes with just a hand in the cot. After 4 am when they wake they do sometimes ask for milk, but they will settle. Often they are awake before 6 am and we will watch the clock change to the sun and then wake up the milk! I'm getting more sleep than before and feel optimistic seeing the progress we have made, while staying true to our principles of gentle parenting."

You might be wondering… "Isn't it a problem substituting my boob for something else? How will I then wean my child off of the back rub, lying down with them or singing to them?" You had a baby who has now grown into a toddler, and now you have successfully weaned him from breastfeeding at night. That does not mean he has outgrown the need to have you there with him, comforting him, and settling him. Research shows that providing your baby with cuddles does not create bad habits, but actually helps children. It builds their neural pathways, enabling them to deal with stress and calm themselves.[2] The older your child gets,

---

2. Cassidy J. Emotion regulation: Influences of attachment relationships. *Monographs of the Society for Research in Child Development.* 1994; 59, 228-283.

the easier it is for him to settle and go to sleep on his own. When my child was ready and I was totally over the whole dragged-out night-time routine, I said, "For the next two nights I will sing to you, but then I'm going to stop doing that." Third night, I said good night and that was it. He was older and totally understood that the singing to bed nights were over! No tears involved at all.

Idea #2 Set up their own bed.

This can be in your room or their own room. If it's easier you can have a room of mattresses as your bedroom. This makes for easier bedsharing/musical beds during the night and for transitioning children out of your bed. This can be the answer. You can also put a toddler mattress next to your bed. This is what my husband and I have done for our three boys. This way they can start out in their own bed and have their own space. It also makes for an easier transition when you are doing idea #1. Now they are being put to sleep in their own bed, without boob. This can help start the night-weaning transition and getting them into their own beds. I know someone who gradually moved their kid's bed farther and farther away from their own bed until eventually it was moved out of their room. Remember, COMMUNICATION WITH THEM IS KEY. Talk to them! They are little humans who understand more than many of us realize…

Idea #3 Have your partner/helper settle your toddler when he wakes in the middle of the night looking for boob.

If you start doing idea #1 and have some success with it, this is an extension of that. Let me note here… when my husband and I started doing this with our middle boy, I remember a couple of times saying to him, "OK, this is the plan tonight. When he wakes up, you cuddle him and try to shoosh him back to sleep." The first few times my husband tried this, our son SCREAMED! Needless to say, I said to my husband, "Forget it! Give him to me!" I breastfed him to sleep. Eventually though, this did work! Two steps forward… one step back. If it does not work today, that does not mean it won't work tomorrow or next week. If you are a sole parent, this is where having your mum/friend/sister sleep over for a few nights and help will really be the support you need to push through!

Idea #4 Be open to the idea of bedsharing without breastfeeding.

After our first-born started going to sleep without boob, he would still wake in the middle of the night, walk down the hall and crawl into our bed. I was totally fine with this because I could actually settle him straight back to sleep without breastfeeding him and I didn't have to get out of bed. If you find that this is not working for you, then put a mattress on the floor next to your bed or get a single bed and push it next to yours. I also know of people who just put their double mattress on the floor with a single one next to it for this purpose, or who bought a king sized bed. Eventually we transitioned our son into his own bed on the floor next to ours and then, all of a sudden a couple of years later, he starting sleeping through the night in his own bed. Remember, those of us living in Western countries are the weird ones of the world. Many families sleep together in the same room! I'm going to venture out here and say that other cultures do this not only because of space issues, but also because it keeps all the kids and babies happy.

Idea #5 Transition your child into his own mattress while talking about "no boobie until the sun comes up" or "boobie until I count to ten."

For our middle boy we had a toddler mattress next to ours and communicated that there was no boobie until the sun came up. For the first couple of nights he would sit up in his own bed, yell out, "Sun up! sun up!" at 3 am in the PITCH dark and try to breastfeed. I would tell him, "No, the sun is not up, go back to sleep" and my husband would shoosh him back to sleep (the mattress was away from me on my husband's side of the bed). Eventually he stopped waking and would wake at the FIRST

BARELY VISIBLE RAY OF SUNSHINE to have boob. You can also use the counting trick for limiting the amount of time your child stays on the breast. This can help with the overall weaning process during the day. Obviously he has to be awake for the counting one!

Idea #6 Cuddle, comfort and talk to your child when they wake.

If you are on your own without help or know that you will be the only person who is able to play the roll of settler, then have no worries! It can be you (the breastfeeding mother) who can do the settling and comforting when your child wakes. Even if you have some help (a partner or family member who can help), you might find that doing it yourself works best.

Idea #7 If you have other children, put them together in the same room.

Often times if they have a sibling to sleep near, a child will feel much more comfortable. With our middle boy, we found that after he night-weaned, he was much easier to transition out of our room , by putting him in the same room as his brother. To this day he loves sharing a room. Of course my oldest, who is almost twelve and acts about sixteen, is not so

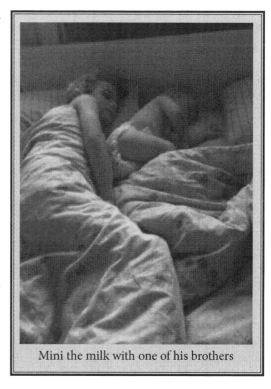

Mini the milk with one of his brothers

keen on the idea of sharing a room with his younger annoying brothers.

Idea #8 Sometimes people have to go to extreme measures to get their toddlers to night-wean.

My dear friend Elle is an example of this. Her second born was an extremely high-needs child. He cried unless he was being held or breastfed. As he got older he would breastfeed FREQUENTLY at night. When I say frequently, I mean he would hardly sleep at all unless he was latched on. She continued to breastfeed him throughout the night while pregnant with her third, and also after she had her baby. Yet her breaking point came a few months after her baby was born. Her breastfeeding toddler was crying so often for boob during the night she could not cope! She was breastfeeding a newborn and trying to settle her three-year-old at the same time. She ended up having to go to a different room with her infant at night, leaving her three-year-old with her partner. Every time he woke up, his dad would try to settle him back to sleep. There were lots of tears from her little boy BUT the crucial difference between this and trying night-weaning with an eight-month-old is that he understood what was going on. He could understand what his dad was telling him, he could understand that he was not alone and he could talk and explain what he was feeling! It is a very different situation doing this with a baby who cannot communicate in any way except to cry and is not developmentally ready to sleep for extended periods of time.

Your child will NOT breastfeed through the night forever. Your child will NOT share your bed or room forever. You will NOT be co-sleeping and breastfeeding your child as they head off to college as many non-supportive people like to speculate will happen. Listen to your child. They will let you know what ideas are working for them—if you have to slow down what you are doing or if you can keep going full-steam ahead. Have flexibility and patience. It is possible to night-wean gently if you continue to be mindful of this.

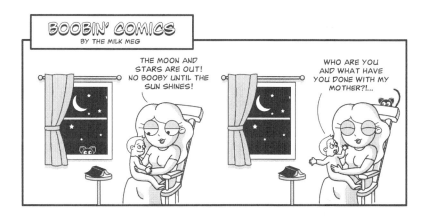

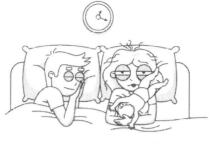

Getting Your Kids Out of Your Bed

"Never let your baby into your bed! You'll never get them out!"

Have you heard that one before? I did many times as a new mother. My husband and I were still in college at the time—the first of our friends to have a baby. We were completely clueless about all things baby. Breastfeeding was going well for me, but one thing that I struggled with was sleep! Every single time I would put my newborn in his little bassinet he would cry. Then I would cry. So the steps from baby in the next room, to co-sleeping (having him in our room), and bedsharing (having him in our bed) went something like this…

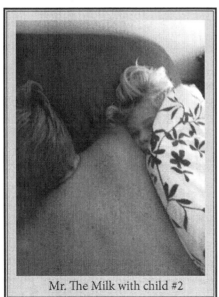

Mr. The Milk with child #2

1. Put baby into the bassinet in the next room. The designated baby room with changing table, bassinet, and breastfeeding chair.

2. Wake up NUMEROUS times throughout the night, pick up baby, breastfeed baby in said breastfeeding chair, change baby, breastfeed again, put baby

back into his bassinet.

3. Cry from utter exhaustion.

4. Half an hour to two hours later repeat steps 1-3.

5. Cry from utter exhaustion. Consider bottle feeding or hiring a wet nurse.

6. Bring bassinet next to bed.

7. Pick up baby, breastfeed in bed, put baby back in bassinet.

8. Cry from utter exhaustion.

9. Half an hour to one hour later repeat step 5-8.

10. Say to husband, "That's it!! He won't sleep unless he is with me! I won't sleep unless he is with me! He needs to come into bed!"

11. Husband says with raised eyebrows, "OK! We will try it."

12. Husband falls back into a deep sleep and does not wake for the next eight hours.

13. Mum wakes frequently but is able to pop out the boob, latch on the baby and fall back to sleep within ten seconds. Bliss.

I know that many of us bring our babies into bed because we find that they sleep longer and/or are more settled and often times we can just pop our boob out without having to even wake up. We do not question that it feels right, we question whether it's the right thing to do because we have no idea how we will stop doing it. My husband and I had no idea how the process of getting our son out of the bed would actually work. If we can have a bit of a plan in place early on so we know how to go about doing this in the future, we can relax a bit and really enjoy co-sleeping (sleeping with our babies right next to us) or bedsharing (having them in our bed with us).

We have three kids now, who all slept in our bed when they were little. We used similar steps for each of them but what worked for one, did not necessarily work for the other! All three of them slept with us from when they were born until they were about 2 years old. This is how we transitioned them from our bed to their own beds...

Baby #1

1. When baby #1 was about two years old my husband started to put him to sleep for the night in his own bed, in his own room. He was used to falling asleep while breastfeeding, so someone from a La Leche League meeting suggested that I try having someone else put him to bed. This way he would not associate sleep with breastfeeding. It worked like magic! My husband would sing to him and lie down with him. He soon started sleeping without breastfeeding. He also completely weaned a few months after I night-weaned him.

2. At some point in the night he would then toddle down the hall and hop into our bed. I would say, "No boobie until the sun comes up" and he would fall back to sleep with us. He slept half the night in his bed and half the night in our bed for about one year, until I was pregnant with baby #2.

3. At this point we felt as though we wanted our first born to be comfortable NOT being in our bed for half the night before the new baby came. We needed more space. It is important to note that many women do sleep four (or more) in a bed and that works just fine for them. It's about doing what feels comfortable for you and your other family members. Happy to cuddle toddler

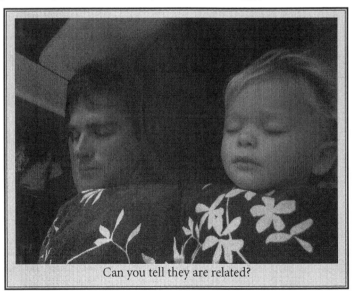
Can you tell they are related?

in one arm and baby in the other? Great! Do what works for you and trust your own instincts on how to go ahead with the sleeping/bedsharing situation.

4. To transition him out of our bed we put a little mattress down on the floor next to our bed and when he woke up he would lie down next to us on his own mattress. He did not like this very much at first, but he was 3 years old at that point and could understand when we told him it was time he slept in his own bed. Communicating with your child is extremely important while doing this. I would put my arm over the side of my bed and he would hold my hand while he fell back to sleep.

5. He ended up waking in the night and sleeping in our room, on his own little mattress next to our bed until he was 5 years old. We would not even wake when he came into our room. He knew he could come in at any time and was comforted being close to us. When we moved from the USA to Australia he magically started sleeping through the night in his own bed! We have no idea why—he was obviously just ready to do it.

Baby #2

Our second baby was the easiest, most chilled-out baby in the history of babies. This child breastfed to sleep happily and easily every day for 3 ½ years. He night-weaned and transitioned into his own bed really quickly and easily.

1. When we started to transition him out of our bed we began in the same way. My husband tried to settle him and put him to bed instead of me when he turned 2 years old. This DID. NOT. WORK. Failed miserably! He really wanted (and needed) to be breastfed to sleep still. So instead, I still breastfed him to sleep but then I would put him on his own mattress (next to our bed) and when he woke we would say, "No boobie until the sun comes up."

2. Once the sun came up he would hop into our bed and breastfeed. He very quickly transitioned into his own bed without waking to get into our bed. He was quite happy in there!

3. We kept his bed next to our bed for about six months. Once he was about 3 years old he started to sleep in his brother's room. He loved being with his older brother and never woke up in the middle of the night to come into our bed. He was happy to be with his big brother and they felt comfortable and safe in their bunk beds.

4. He breastfed until he was 3 ½ years old but from 2 to 3 ½ he did not breastfeed throughout the night and did not sleep in our bed.

Baby #3

Baby #2 was chill, easy, and relaxed. Baby #3 (otherwise known as "Mini The Milk") has never been chill, easy, or relaxed about sleep! He has pretty much hated sleep since the day he was born. Do you have one of these?!

1. From when he was about a year old, we put a little toddler bed next to our bed, which I would put him in to start with when he first fell asleep. After he woke to breastfeed I would either put him back (or try to put him back) in his bed. He spent some of the night in our bed and some of the night in his bed (depending on how frequently he woke and if he was settled or not).

2. From when he was about 20 months old, we started having my husband put him to sleep in the baby carrier instead of me breastfeeding him to sleep. However, he still woke ALL THE TIME to breastfeed!

3. Although he would fall asleep with my husband while being carried, he was still waking very frequently at night and would not resettle in his own bed easily. After MANY EXHAUSTING, ANNOYING, TEARS-STREAMING-DOWN-MY-CHEEKS NIGHTS, I knew that we needed to night-wean and transition him into his own bed 100% so he and I could sleep! Although he would not resettle easily in his own bed, he was not a cuddler. He would always breastfeed and then roll away from me as far as possible! He wanted to be with us but not touching us. At all!

4. At the age of 2 ½ we successfully night-weaned him. We quickly realized that after the first two nights of being glued to my husband, he actually really wanted to be sleeping on his own! He would settle much more quickly when in his own space. My husband would talk to him about "no boobie until the sun comes up" and would then comfort him with a hand on his back or with a little song, all while he was in his own bed next to our bed. Did he like this plan? No! He thrashed around, cried and had a tantrum, however he was 2 ½, developmentally able to understand what we were saying, and he could explain his feelings. We talked to him, cuddled him (when he wanted it) and we were there for him at every step of the way. It took about one week for him to sleep through the night. Nights two and three were the hardest, but he had us there with him throughout it all.

5. He slept in our room, in his own bed for about two months. After that time (when we knew he was sleeping through), we moved him into his big boy bed in a room with his older brother. He loves his new bed. At the time of writing this, he is 2 ½ years old and my husband still carries him in the baby carrier to fall asleep, or sometimes I breastfeed him to sleep and then we put him down in his room. Don't get me wrong… the second that ray of sunshine is there he is up, toddling to our room asking for "boobies!"

Some key points about transitioning your child out of your bed…

Siblings. If there is an older sibling that they share a room with, the transition can go much more smoothly. I mean, who wants to sleep all alone?! We are social creatures. Most adults prefer to sleep with someone at least in the same room as us so we are not alone at night. Babies, toddlers, and children are the same.

It does not happen overnight. If you can be open to the idea that this will take time and not happen overnight, you can avoid your child becoming distressed, crying by herself, or needing to hire a sleep consultant. Just trust your instincts and follow your child's lead. Be gentle and allow it to happen gradually, in steps.

Communicate. Communicate with your child as much as possible about the new bed or why you need some more space at night. Children are quite amazing in how much they understand and can appreciate where you are coming from. Be honest and be a good communicator.

Respect where your child is at, even if it doesn't work for you. Some kids will respond really quickly to the transition and others won't. Respect your child's feelings, along with your own feelings and your partner's feelings.

Consider a room of mattresses. I know quite a few families who have a room of mattresses on the floor or a room of mattresses on metal bed frames! For Mini The Milk (baby #3) my husband put a toddler bed frame on stilts so it was in line with our bed. I promise you… once your children get older, the last thing they will want to do is sleep in the same room as you. My eleven-year-old (baby #1) would be horrified if he had to sleep in our room! Funny how things change.

The connection between breastfeeding and bedsharing or co-sleeping. Many parents find that their babies or toddlers do not happily sleep on their own until they are night-weaned. However, there are always exceptions. My mother breastfed me during the night for over a year but I always happily slept in my own cot in my own room. Night-weaning can be done without much stress or heartache once your child is nearing the 18-month mark. This is because most toddlers at this age can understand what you are saying. You can communicate with your child and have a conversation about night-weaning and/or moving him into his own bed, regardless of whether it is in your room or in his own room.

Trust your instincts, go gently, and be patient. Our three boys have been breastfed on demand, cuddled all night by us, co-slept, bedshared and we never had them self-settle. All three of them now sleep in their own beds and through the night. Enjoy the night-time breastfeeds while they last. It's a special time.

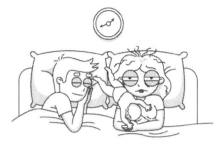

Frequent Breastfeeding and Cavities

"I was told by my dentist that I have to night-wean my child. Is this true?"

"I was told that frequent breastfeeding is the cause of my child's dental issues."

I cannot write a book about how it's biologically normal for your breastfed children to be waking at night without discussing cavities, since I receive questions about this almost daily from people. I do need to start with what first comes to my mind… It makes absolutely no sense whatsoever from an anthropological or evolutionary perspective that something so common and biologically normal (breastfeeding throughout the night) would lead to cavities. We have survived as a species because what happens naturally works pretty well most of the time! Birthing, breastfeeding, and sleeping with or close to our babies has worked since the beginning of human existence.

Biological anthropologist Gwen Dewar, PhD, wrote, "Hunter-gatherer babies nurse very frequently—twice an hour or more."[1] This frequent breastfeeding is of course not only during the day, but also during the night as well. While our babies do tend to space out their feedings as they get older, many mothers find

1. Dewar, G. Breastfeeding on demand. *Parenting Science*. http://www.parentingscience.com/breastfeeding-on-demand.html. Published 2008. Modified February 2014. Accessed May 12, 2014.

that they continue to breastfeed frequently at times, including during the night. It is not logical that the behaviour many of us experience in following the lead of our babies would be destroying their teeth. The most current research also supports this! There is NO evidence-based, good, solid research out there that shows cavities are caused by breastfeeding.

There is no evidence to suggest that breastfeeding or its duration are independent risk factors for early childhood caries, severe early childhood caries, or decayed and filled surfaces on primary teeth.[2] Antibodies in breastmilk help to impede bacterial growth (including Streptococcus mutans, which is the bacterium that causes tooth decay).[3] As dentist Brian Palmer wrote, "Human milk alone does not cause dental caries. Infants exclusively breastfed are not immune to decay due to other factors that impact the infant's risk for tooth decay. Decay causing bacteria (Streptococcus mutans) is transmitted to the infant by way of parents, caregivers, and others."[4]

The antibodies in breastmilk inhibit the growth of cavity-causing bacteria including Streptococcus mutans. A protein in breastmilk called lactoferrin actually kills it.[5] Research tells us that the following DO contribute to cavities: sugar, formula, poor diet, family genetics, and dental hygiene.

What's the take-home message? Current evidence-based research shows that breastfeeding at night does NOT cause cavities and that the opposite is actually true: breastmilk helps protect teeth. Also, breastmilk does not pool in a baby's mouth as many people think. The nipple is pulled very far back while

2. Lida H, Auinger P, Billings R, Weitzman M. A bactericidal effect for human lactoferrin. *Pediatrics.* 2007; 120 no. 4 e944-e952. doi: 10.1542/peds.2006-0124

3. Arnold R, Cole M, McGhee J. A bactericidal effect for human lactoferrin. *Science.* 1997; 197:263–65.

4. Palmer D. Breastfeeding and infant caries: No connection. *The Newsletter of The Academy of Breastfeeding Medicine.* 2000; 6 no. 4, 27–31.

5. Mandel ID. Caries prevention: current strategies, new directions. *JADA.* 1996; 127:1477–88.

breastfeeding. While breastmilk does not collect in a baby's mouth, bottled breastmilk or formula does. Putting your baby to bed with a bottle is NOT advised, regardless of what is in the bottle.

If you are happily breastfeeding at night, instead of focusing on unnecessary weaning, look at the many other factors that contribute to cavities and see what dietary/lifestyle changes you can make… and keep on boobin'!

TAKE THE TIME TO JUST
SIT AND HANG OUT WITH
YOUR BABY SKIN-TO-
SKIN. OFTEN TIMES THIS
IS ALL THEY NEED.
FREQUENT CUDDLES AND
FREQUENT BOOBIN'.

SKIN-TO-SKIN
CHANGE OF SCENERY
CUDDLES

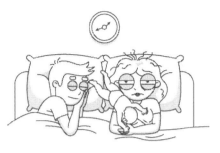

Tips to Settle Your Baby...
When Boob Doesn't Work

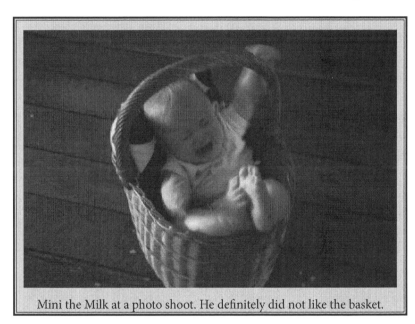

Mini the Milk at a photo shoot. He definitely did not like the basket.

Is it colic? Is he allergic to something in my milk? What is happening?!

In this book I write frequently about breastfeeding for comfort, breastfeeding to sleep, and whipping a boob out whenever your baby is cranky. However, there will definitely be times when breastfeeding just does not work! This chapter will go over some tips for you and the circuit, which is a collection of suggestions to help settle your baby.

You have tried it all… breastfeeding, rocking, pacing the halls, passing him back and forth, crying , sitting, standing, tearing your hair out, and he is still crying! What is a mother to do? We all have the same fundamental question: "Is my baby normal?" Is it normal for my baby to be cranky, to breastfeed constantly, to only sleep when I'm carrying him, etc. etc. etc…. and the reality is, yes! It is normal for your baby to be cranky at times for no apparent reason. Does that make you feel better or worse? I remember my mother calling the hours in the later afternoon the "witching hour." You know that time when you have your baby on your hip or in a sling while trying to make dinner, sweep up all the crumbs off the floor, put that last load of laundry in, and try to get one piece of food in your mouth before you starve to death?

Before I had children I had all of these ideas as to what parenthood would be like. Remember before you had children? That distant past that seems blurry now due to your sleep deprivation? Remember looking at those other parents as a young twenty year old thinking, "Wow, when I'm a parent, I will NEVER do that! How horrible!" Yet now you find yourself doing that same exact thing… this is what happens! No one imagines themselves looking at their baby thinking, "Why are you so cranky?! I'm a horrible parent, I can't even settle my own baby!" Yet, these are thoughts we all have from time to time. It's normal.

Every month when I have my Boobies By the Beach group meet-up (a breastfeeding group for mums to get together and chat about all things breastfeeding) nearly every time there's a wonderful moment when someone will hear a mother's story and say, "My baby does that too! Oh good, it's normal!" This is especially important for issues regarding normal breastfeeding behavior, sleep, and cranky babies. Hearing that someone else has a baby that does the same thing as your baby creates an instant feeling of relief.

From my own experiences (and talking with many women over the past nine years since having my first-born, very high needs, cranky baby) I have learned a thing or two about crankiness… there is light at the end of this long dark cranky tunnel! One of my friends coined the term, "the circuit" as a way to describe what she did when her babies were upset. The idea is that you keep going through the list until, voila, the baby stops crying! You will then fall into a heap on the couch and cry yourself to sleep from happiness that your baby is finally content.

1. Breastfeed your baby. When in doubt, whip it out! Always my go-to-step! Although this doesn't always work…

2. Carry your baby… on your hip, in a sling, hanging like a star fish in a Baby Bjorn, however you want to do it! Just carry them. Many babies like to breastfeed while being walked around in a sling. One of my friends had to breastfeed her baby while walking ALL THE TIME. It's amazing her legs didn't fall off. Come to think of it, she looks extremely fit and healthy and this could be the reason why. It's a great way to get some exercise! Some babies just need this extra movement to settle.

3. Get skin to skin with your baby. The power of skin-to-skin is often times underestimated.

4. Pass your baby to your husband, partner, friend, neighbor, random stranger in the park (just kidding!) so you can get a break. You will feel better knowing that although they are crying, at least they are being held.

5. Go for a walk outside with your baby and put them in a pram/stroller/baby carrier. Sometimes just a change in scenery is enough.

6. Get into the bath with your baby. You can also try breastfeeding in the bath. Some babies love it.

7. Back to step one!

…And around and around it goes until eventually one of these steps will work. Of course if one of these just isn't feeling right for you or your baby then skip it. Also, add whatever else you can think of to the list.

Even after having my third I would still think, "But I just breastfed you five minutes ago!" before putting him back on the boob. Yet I know that often babies will do this. They will pull off, get cranky, want to be walked around and then five minutes later get back on the breast and fall asleep happily. What is the deal!? Well, they have a biological need to be with their mothers and breastfeed A LOT. I think it's helpful to know that it's normal, and you'll get through this long dark cranky tunnel.

A baby's unsettled behavior can also be due to a tongue or lip tie. However in these cases there are often quite a few different symptoms happening at the same time (baby has difficulty feeding, reflux symptoms, mother has damaged nipples, etc.) and these will happen at various times both during the day and at night. Seek help if you suspect this might be the problem.

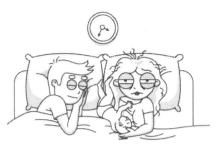

Gut Health, Food Intolerance and Abnormal Night-Waking

Now that you have read all of the reasons frequent night-waking is totally normal, it's important for me to acknowledge that there are of course circumstances where it's not! If your child's frequent night-waking is not due to teething pain, developmental milestones, or needing some comfort, it might be due to medical or health issues that can be helped! There are different examples of health issues that can affect sleep, but the one I will go over is one of the most common causes of colic symptoms (an unsettled baby, unexplained weight loss or slow gain, rashes/eczema): food intolerances.

*An intolerance is different from an allergy. An allergy to a particular food causes an immune system reaction within your body, affects organs, and can be life-threatening. Intolerance to a food usually has less severe symptoms and sometimes people can tolerate small amounts of the food (especially after having eliminated it for an extended period of time) without having any symptoms or may only experience mild discomfort.

I am extremely passionate about gut health and could write an entire book on it (maybe I will some day! Possibly when I am not breastfeeding, pregnant, or sleep deprived!). The bacteria present (or not present) within our digestive tract can be the underlying cause of many digestive issues, including food intolerances.

One interesting study on bacteria and allergies in children found that, "Increased bacterial diversity in infants' intestinal flora reduced risk of allergic sensitization, allergic rhinitis, and peripheral blood eosinophilia.

Although a particular bacterial strain was not found to be protective, results suggest that certain pathogenic bacteria such as Staphylococcus sp. may increase risk for allergic disease, possibly through reduction in diversity of intestinal flora."[1]

Here are some main points to remember about gut health (the health of our digestive system):

Your gut flora is made up of microorganisms that live within your digestive system. These include bacteria and fungi and affect all aspects of our health and immune system. "Dynamic balances exist between the gastrointestinal microbiota, host physiology, and diet that directly influence the initial acquisition, developmental succession, and eventual stability of the gut ecosystem."[2] One researcher stated, "Our study indicates that flora with a diet dependent pattern is already present in the first days of life."[3] Gut flora is what helps us break down and digest our food. If we do not have a healthy, functioning gut, then we may have trouble tolerating some foods.

Although there is much that is misunderstood about allergies and food intolerances, it is clear that babies who are susceptible to allergies can be affected by a single exposure to the protein in cow's milk. This can disrupt the lining of the gut and create an inflammatory response, which then leads to an intolerance or allergy for the baby.

1. Bisgaard H, Li N, Donnelykke K. Reduced diversity of the intestinal microbiota during infancy is associated with increased risk of allergic disease at school age. *J Allergy Clin Immunol.* 2011; 128(3):646–652

2. Mackie R, Sghir A, Gaskins R. Developmental microbial ecology of the neonatal gastrointestinal tract. *American Society for Clinical Nutrition.* 1999; 69(5):1035s–1045s.

3. Rubaltelli F, Biadaioli R, Pecile P, Nicoletti P. Intestinal flora in breast- and bottle-fed infants. *J Perinat Med.* 1998; 26(3):186–91.

"Exclusive consumption of breastmilk facilitates the early maturation of the intestinal barrier and provides a passive barrier to potentially antigenic molecules until the baby's own natural barriers develop."[4]

So while breastfeeding creates a protective barrier, for babies with an extreme sensitivity to dairy in their mother's milk (from their mother consuming cow's milk products), this barrier might not be enough to prevent symptoms of intolerances or allergies. Gluten, soy, corn, and nuts are other common foods that babies can have an intolerance to.

Some symptoms of food intolerances include nervousness, tremor, sweating, palpitations, rapid breathing, headache, migraine, diarrhea, burning sensations on the skin, tightness across the face and chest, breathing problems ,asthma-like symptoms, and allergy-like reactions.[5] It is no wonder then that our children's sleep can be affected if they are experiencing some of these symptoms!

I always suggest to women that they eliminate dairy first, as I have found while working with women that this is the most common food that can cause problems while breastfeeding. It must be cut out 100% though (not even in a cracker!) and it's not just a matter of having lactose free milk as it's not the lactose in many cases, but rather the actual protein in the dairy. If dairy is not the culprit, then I suggest trying gluten next.

4. Riordann J. *Breastfeeding and human lactation.* 4th ed. Boston, NY: Jones and Bartlett Publishers; 2010.

5. Allergy and intolerance. NSW Food Authority. http://www.foodauthority. nsw.gov.au/consumers/problems-with-food/allergy-and-intolerance#. VPZY_fmUeSo. Updated July 2014. Accessed December 9, 2014.

Here is Holly's experience with her child's sleep and the connection between gluten and his unsettled behavior during the night:

> From the time Leo was born, there was no rhythm to his sleep patterns. By day he was a wonderfully happy baby, but at night there was no telling how many times or for how long he (we) would be awake. Every night was different and some nights he was extremely agitated and inconsolable. He wasn't interested in breastfeeding (though always available) and there was total inconsistency in timing and extreme unhappiness... paired with the experience of our first child sleeping through the night from 8 months until there was a sibling ... so there was obviously a concern based on the contrast. I have since realized that in most situations contrasting behaviours don't at all indicate an issue, just different personalities. Not always so with the sleep situation.
>
> We visited our naturopathic midwife (NPMW) when Leo was about 18 months old. She immediately thought of food sensitivity and it turned out gluten was our culprit. It only took a few months to see noted improvements, but it took a good 12–18 months of no gluten to see the full effects. Finally though, there was consistent sleep. I will also note that our NPMW also realized I needed to sleep for my health and so worked with me on relaxation and aromatherapy while we were working on craniosacral treatments with Leo. Now he is 8 and every now and then after he goes to sleep I recall the sense of anxiousness we lived with not knowing if he would stay asleep for 5 minutes or 5 hours or anywhere in between... it is amazing how our systems can react... AND recover!

*Interesting side note... Leo now eats gluten with no effects ... When I omitted gluten from my diet for a year or more because I was breastfeeding, I noted lots of amazing improvements in skin health and decreased discomforts in many areas of my health. I continue to eat a mainly gluten free diet and continue to see the benefits!

All of the awesome bacteria that are in our bodies pass through our breastmilk to our children.[6] Therefore, it's important to not only continue breastfeeding while going through an elimination diet, but to also work on the microbes within your gut, so all of the goodness can go to your child.

Seek help from an International Board Certified Lactation Consultant and/or other health care professionals with knowledge about breastfeeding, food intolerances, gut health, and infant feeding. Diet and rebuilding your gut health (with probiotics found in capsules and fermented and cultured foods) are equally important. We have over 100 trillion bacteria in our bodies right now with an estimated 10,000 different strains of bacteria! It's estimated that the bacteria within our bodies weigh 0.5-1.3kg (1-3 pounds)! It is imperative that we pay close attention to this through what we are eating. Let's get back to how humans have always eaten: a diet rich in whole foods, fermented foods, and cultured foods. Every culture in the world has a history of a fermented or cultured food product within their regular diets. Now get out there and eat some sauerkraut!

6   Ted J, Christophe L, Christian B, Florence R, Christophe C. Vertical mother–neonate transfer of maternal gut bacteria via breastfeeding. *Environmental Microbiology.* 2013; 16 (9):2891–2904. doi: 10.1111/1462-2920.12238

NO MOTHER LOOKS
BACK AND FEELS
GUILTY FOR CUDDLING
OR BREASTFEEDING
HER BABY TOO OFTEN.
YOU CANNOT SPOIL A
BABY. YOU CANNOT
CUDDLE THEM TOO
OFTEN. BREASTFEED
THEM TOO FREQUENTLY.
OR LOVE THEM
TOO MUCH. ♥

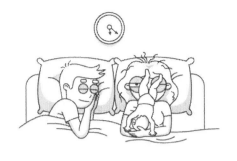

As Your Child Grows...

At the time of writing my oldest boy is eleven years old. I remember his birth so well. I remember his first breastfeed, the first time I decided to bring him into bed with us, and the first time he slept in his big boy bed and then toddled into our room at midnight to hop into our bed. All of these moments that felt so incredibly intense at the time are now memories. He does not breastfeed anymore. He does not fall asleep in my arms or reach for me during the night. He does not call out for me to ask for "booby." He falls asleep on his own, puts his headphones in, asks to sleep over at friends' houses and barely says goodbye as he leaves the house. He is growing up, but he still needs me sometimes in ways that surprise me.

During his early childhood years, between about 5 and 7, he would wake sometimes with night terrors. I would sit with him until he relaxed or we would bring him into bed with us. I remember one of the only times he had an ear infection. He was about 6 years old and woke crying and complaining that his ear hurt. We brought him into our room and set up a little mattress on the floor so he could lie on it for the night. I could monitor how he was doing and easily check on him and he could also ask for my help if he needed it, without yelling down the hall.

Just recently he woke me up in the middle of the night, "I had a bad dream!" He was really distressed and I knew it must have been a terrible dream for him to walk all the way to our room since he had not done that in about 5 years! I asked if he wanted to sleep in our room and he immediately said, "Yes!" He got his blanket and pillow and set up the little mattress on the floor next to our bed, just as he had done when he was a little boy.

The need to be in close proximity to other humans is not something that we grow out of. Our children stop waking to breastfeed, they stop waking for a cuddle, they sleep through the night… yet even those of us who are grown and independent still need someone to turn to at 2am sometimes. We feel scared, we feel alone, and we feel the need for comfort. Comfort is something that we give our babies, our toddlers, and our growing children. We give this to adults, to family, and to friends. It starts as mothering through breastfeeding and continues as mothering through comfort in many different forms. Feel confident in mothering through breastfeeding and cuddling during the day and at night, just as nature intended. Feel confident in continuing to comfort your child at night when they wake. These moments go from breastfeeds to just simply allowing them the opportunity to be near you. You will never look back and regret being there for them when they needed it most.

KEEP
ON
BOOBIN'

Trust your instincts.

Follow the lead of your baby.

And of course...

Keep on boobin'.

-The Milk Meg
Meg Nagle, IBCLC

Find Meg on Facebook and all social media sites!
Search "The Milk Meg."

Visit Meg's website/blog: www.themilkmeg.com

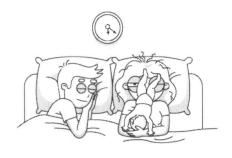